A CLASSICAL VET IN
MODERN TIMES

Best
wishes

Richard B
May 2005

A CLASSICAL VET IN MODERN TIMES

R Llewellyn Brown

ATHENA PRESS
LONDON

A CASSICAL VET IN MODERN TIMES
Copyright © R Llewellyn Brown 2005

ISBN 1 84401 330 8

First Published 2005 by
ATHENA PRESS
Queen's House, 2 Holly Road
Twickenham TW1 4EG
United Kingdom

Printed for Athena Press

For Heather, Rebecca and Phillip.

With grateful thanks to the *Veterinary Times*, who have published small sections of this book in the past.

Acknowledgements

I would like to acknowledge the encouragement given to me by three people: Lydia Brown, Elizabeth Buchanan and David Watson have, at various times, suggested I put pen to paper. They are of course in no way responsible for the faults in this book.

Chapter One

We are such stuff as dreams are made on ...

The Tempest, William Shakespeare

'He says the bull isn't here.' Xavier, my veterinary assistant, turned round from the Mennonite farmer and looked at me. His face, typical of a Mayan Indian, displayed no emotion apart from a thin smile. I got out of my Land Rover and took a pace along the recently-cut guinea grass that passed for a lawn. Between the tussocks I could see the bright red earth and the occasional black ant scurrying along, busy to complete its task. I stopped a few yards short of the group of three: Xavier, the Mennonite farmer and his son.

'What does he mean? Is it dead or what?' I queried, looking at the farmer. The strong Belizean sun reflected off his wide-brimmed hat. He stood with his arms hanging loosely by his side, while next to him his teenage son chewed away at some grass. I looked over and behind them to his wooden house, a mixture of American, Mennonite and Amish in style. The door was open but only revealed a mosquito net curtain door. The windows had louvres, but again a mosquito net was behind them and one could hardly make out the plain patterned cotton curtains. Typically for Central America, the house appeared a little dilapidated at the edges. The paint was chipped, and an odd nail loose. The tropical storms and searing heat had eventually weathered everything. Clothes lines ran from the house over angled poles to nearby trees. A few plain shirts, blouses and dungarees hung on them. I could just see, hiding behind the house, the Mennonite's wife and daughters, engaged in domestic chores. Now and then one of them sneaked a look at Xavier, the Mayan Indian, or me, the British Veterinary Officer.

The farmer mumbled something. I couldn't make it out.

Xavier turned and smiled broadly, revealing his perfect teeth. He had a wicked sense of humour and appeared to be enjoying the joke.

'He says the bull is miles away in the middle of the jungle. If you want to read the test for tuberculosis, you are going to have to go in there yourself.' He smirked, keeping his face away from the Mennonites and came close to me, brushing his feet against the rough grass.

'Xavier, did he say *read* the test? Has he got training?' I asked in doubt. Belize was always full of surprises. Perhaps the Mennonite *did* know about the TB test, and how you had to come back three days later and check the size of lumps at the sites in the skin where I had injected the tuberculin antigen.

'No, no, boss.' Xavier was enjoying himself immensely now. 'Calm yourself. He just said "test", not "*read* the test". *Probar*. I just changed it for you to the correct English. *Probar*, Spanish – to test.'

'Thank you for the Spanish, Xavier.' My spoken Spanish was average and I couldn't always understand Spanish with a Mennonite tinge. 'How come he is the only one who hasn't kept his animal in ready for us to check a few days later? We've spent all day checking the new imports of all his neighbours and they all kept their bulls and cows handy.' I nodded over my shoulder to the square miles of cleared bush behind me. Dotted across these rolling hillocks were similar Mennonite farmhouses interspersed by tracks, fences and fields with a smattering of livestock. Each one was a family farm.

'I don't know, boss, but be very careful. This farmer here is a Ziegler. Some people say they are involved in drugs and guns and so on.' Xavier was speaking down to the ground as much as to me.

'Okay, okay, Xavier. I take the point. Still, we have to check this bull. See if he can help us a bit,' I suggested.

'Right, boss.' Xavier smiled and turned to the Mennonite and ambled toward him. Xavier's face suddenly became serious as he took on his role of government servant. He shot out some sentences and pointed to the jungle, which was about three quarters of a mile beyond the house. The Mennonite replied and pointed at his son and then at our vehicle and at his old pickup.

Xavier nodded and shook the Mennonite's hand. As far as I could gather I was about to get a lift.

'It is settled. To save our petrol to make sure we get back tonight they will take us in to the jungle to the pen where the bull is. Well, no... The son will take you in and I will stay here and guard the situation.' He nodded at the farmer and our Rover.

'That seems reasonable to me,' I said, and went to the Rover. The metal of the car was hot as I grabbed my testing callipers, book and butterfly net from the back. Lepidoptery was a relaxation which Xavier and others kindly tolerated. The son came up to me in the battered old Ford truck. I got in. Just before we moved off the farmer appeared from nowhere and handed his son a rifle.

'You know what to do with it,' he said clearly.

I was worried not so much by the rifle but by Xavier's expression of concern. This had not been part of our plan. There was not much contest between a butterfly net and a rifle. We lurched off, driving parallel to the edge of the jungle less than a mile away. Deep ditches and barbed-wire fences edged the track. At the first intersection of tracks the son wheeled the car round to the right and headed straight toward the jungle. The trees of the *selva* stood out as a broad, dark green band dividing the blue sky from the light green fields spattered with a few white blobs of cattle in the foreground, all of them white Brahma cows. The pickup went down a slope that consisted of bare smoothed rocks; the entire top surface had been washed away. Once we came down to the same level as the jungle I saw that there was a large gap in the trees on either side of the track. The track was still very bumpy and the American-style springs gave us a rolling sensation as we headed in. We entered the jungle and the sensation was similar to that of continuously entering a large amphitheatre. The tall trees, although far back from the road, gave the impression of being the high walls of the theatre. Their top branches were buttresses which joined the walls to the ceiling in the sky.

I looked at the bushes, many only about three feet tall, on either side of me. All I could see amongst them were the typical common butterflies: pierids, blues, hesperids and so on. There was nothing very special to catch my eye. For interesting butterflies you really needed a fresh jungle clearing with creepers and vines full of flowers writhing over the fallen dead trees. This roadside area had been knocked down some time ago. Suddenly the pickup went very quiet, yet we were still moving. I looked out down to the road and quickly looked back.

Oh no, no, I thought. I looked at the bushes; they were now only one foot high and the track had very subtly widened a foot or two. *I am on a drug trafficker's landing strip…* It was brilliantly disguised and as smooth as glass. Out of the corner of my eye I looked at the son, his rifle leaning on his thigh, the butt propped against the gearstick. I looked dead ahead and prayed. Somewhere I knew there would be three barrels of aviation fuel ready; twenty-four hours a day, three hundred and sixty-five days a year. Some local folk earned their annual income solely by making sure the drug planes could land, refuel, and take off in five minutes. I had seen it myself from a small hill in another district when treating a cow. They had the plane in the air again before I had finished injecting the cow.

Suddenly the noise started again. *Bump, bump, bump.* We were still on the straight track but had just left the runway. Almost immediately on the right we came across the small stockade. It was constructed from trunks of wood that had weathered to a silvery-grey colour. The vertical and horizontal pieces were bolted together. Rust was already beginning to stain the wood below these joins. The top spar was at least six feet high. I alighted from the pickup, made my way carefully through the low bushes, and lifted myself up to get a view inside. The huge Brahma bull was inside the pen with some fodder thrown on the ground for food, a supply of water, and three barrels of aviation fuel.

Few surprises there, I thought to myself. I surveyed the inside. Along one side there was a race, which we could trap him in. The son came beside me.

'We race him in, *ja*?' he queried.

'Fine, but we need a stick or log to put behind him to keep him in while I check him,' I said. 'This,' I pointed to one trunk, 'is too weak, he will smash it with one kick.'

'I know,' said the son and he went round one side of the pen. There were a few very thick mahogany planks lying together. He gestured to them.

'Ideal,' I said, and as he was about to pick one up I shouted, '*Stop!*'

He looked bemused. I flicked it over with my foot: sure enough, a couple of scorpions were hidden there. They scuttled away. Xavier had taught me they often prefer planed mahogany.

'Very good,' said the son, smiling. We kicked a plank to our satisfaction and then lifted it up and over into the pen. 'I know this bull. Just stand behind me always, okay?' he said.

'Fine by me,' I said. I quickly checked my escape routes before I joined him down in the burning hot pen. It has never ceased to surprise me how high you can jump if a bull is really after you. The important point is to make sure the footholds are certain.

'*Tch, tch, tch.*' The son indicated the bull the direction to go. At first the bull swayed his head from side to side. His vast dewlap followed each sideways movement a little late. His eyes were invisible in their dark sockets. Then he began to move in the direction the son suggested.

'Stay behind, stay behind,' the son whispered to me. The bull entered the race but slowly stopped halfway in. We held our breath. The sun beat down on us; reflexly, I licked my lips. Then the bull walked a few more paces and stopped. We shot the mahogany plank in behind him. He was quiet and just stood. It was on the tip of my tongue to say that he must be on drugs or something to be so well behaved. Instead I quickly went round to the side where three days before I had injected him. The clip marks were present just in front of his shoulder hump on the upper neck. The white hair had been clipped away revealing the black skin typical of these zebu types. I felt the skin. There was no thickening in either injection site. He had passed the test.

'Okay. He is clear. He has passed,' I said.

'Good, then I do not need this,' said the son indicating the rifle which I now saw he had put in the pen. 'Only joking! Besides, would I use it on the bull or you? Time to go home, eh? And that barrels, they are for the half-track over there.'

He nodded and I could see through the gaps a bulldozer half immersed in the jungle. I did not know what to believe, but it did seem a good time to go. My job was done. I looked up to the sky as a long-tailed bird flew above us. It landed and I shaded my eyes to catch a view. It was a quetzal, a native of Guetamala straying over the border. Its bright green feathers flashed in the sun. We turned and remounted the pickup. I grimaced at the hot plastic seats.

We travelled back. He could have driven at least eighty mph on the runway, but instead took the pickup at a speed suitable for a rough track. Now the son was humming to himself, all tension gone. He drove up the rise, turned the pickup left at the intersection and headed for the house. I could see another vehicle parked beside my Land Rover, which Xavier had parked under a mango tree to keep it from the heat of the sun. Two men got out, and at the same time the son stopped humming, squinted at the people by his farm and accelerated a little. We arrived and Xavier peeled away from the group of men, all in an animated discussion.

'Clear, boss?' he said.

'Yes, but different. I will tell you later. What's up now – they all look pretty raised up?' I looked at the Mennonite farmer talking tersely to two other Mennonites. Then they pointed at me and looked at me. One asked Xavier something.

'Boss, there is a problem here. It is none of our business, but it is serious. Ziegler's brother has just been found drowned by the dam. He was floating against the dam wall. Also his Rottweiler guard dog was floating beside him. They were seen alive first thing this morning. They ask you to post-mortem the dog. It is a suspicious death and fresh carcase.' Xavier looked noncommittal. 'Perhaps we should do it and report our findings to Ziegler and our superiors?'

'Fresh?' I said. 'Then this must be a dream. The Rottweiler I post-mortemed in Belize was four days gone and full of maggots when we found it by the dam.'

'Yes,' said Xavier, 'this is a dream for sure, boss.' And his face came close to me with a big smile. Just then I felt myself lift away from all those problems, I could see the trees down below me by the farmhouse, Xavier looking up and waving at me and then I was gone. I felt myself drift somewhere else.

This dream must go to somewhere better, I thought, *away from all those fears of physical danger.* I tried to wake myself from the dream. I knew I wanted to return to the real world but could not. I was not in control of what was happening. I wrestled and writhed but still found myself trapped, unable to escape. A little panic set in but then I knew I had moved on.

I felt myself land on a seat. I was back in a classroom, still in a dream. On my left was a large bow window over six yards in width. Each curved pane of glass was at least two and half feet wide and six feet high. Through the glass I could see a small lake a few hundred yards away with a reed bed on the left edge. Opposite on the right bank stood a large copper beech tree. Elsewhere in my view there were wide open spaces with games pitches and occasional clumps of azaleas or bamboos, while to my right I found I was on the edge of a group of twenty-five desks set in a five by five square formation. The chair did not move. I looked down. I was in one of the old-style desks were the metal frame of the chair was in one piece with the frame of the desk table. The wood was old and well polished. In front two blackboards straddled a central desk. The time was five past nine; I recognised my contemporary school students, and the book on my desktop, *Kennedy's Latin Grammar*. The word Latin had, de rigueur, been converted into 'Eating'. *It must be Tuesday morning*, I thought: double Classics until eleven o'clock. Sure enough, the door opened and the Classics master walked in briskly. It was Dr Leasden, his large grey eyebrows turned up at their outer extremities. His slightly tanned skin held a hint of a grin on his face. He examined quickly the occupants of the classroom.

'Good morning, scholars,' he said.

'Good morning, sir,' we all dutifully replied.

'Well, a double lesson today. Time for us to engage fully in the art and science of Classics. With this in mind I think we can commence with some gentle work. Let us begin with simple classical history. After all, on this day some of you may meet your Waterloo.' He looked down at his notes on the desk. At times the desk half hid him. Leasden was not a tall man. 'So, a little light skirmishing. In the second Punic Wars, name me one battle which may seem to the Romans to have been their Waterloo?. Let me see, O'Connor?'

'Trasimene, sir,' replied O'Connor with alacrity.

'Why?' snapped Leasden.

'The consul Flaminius was killed, and possibly as many as 15,000 troops died. The army was annihilated in the mists and confusion by the lake,' added O'Connor.

'Good, I will accept that. Any other similar Waterloos for the Latin race?' A host of hands rose. I was less certain. 'Yes, Burke?'

'Cannae, sir, 216 BC,' said a breathless Burke.

'Good! Now, what possible mistake did Hannibal then make after the battle?' A forest of hands shot up, except mine. I was bemused. Hannibal had smashed the Romans to bits. Was that not enough? It was, after all, what I dreamt of doing to all enthusiasts of Classics – and Hannibal had done it!

'Yes, Seamer…' Leasden turned his gaze to me. 'Jones, I note your tardiness. You are answering the next question.' I gulped and involuntarily squeezed my legs together in the tension. Seamer flowed on.

'Maharbal told Hannibal to immediately march on Rome. Hannibal refused. It was probably his most serious mistake.'

'Fair enough. Now, Jones, what was Hannibal's Waterloo?' I sensed all the class knew. I had only one shot in my locker. The only other battle I could recollect in the whole of the Punic wars.

'Zama, sir,' I pleaded.

'Yes, Jones. No need to be so timorous.'

But then I thought, *He could say that…* He was the cobra. I was the rat. Leasden glided on.

'I won't ask you the date, which for your possible additional intelligence was 202 BC. However, I will ask you the name of the general who defeated Hannibal… Jones?' He raised one eyebrow.

'Scipio Africanus, sir,' I said, a little more certain of my ground.

'Good, proper name, Haslett?' Leasden knew I had not a clue of any fine details.

'Publius Cornelius Scipio,' came the easy reply.

'"Put Hannibal in the scales: how many pounds will that peerless general mark up today? This is the man for whom Africa was too small a continent…" Author, anyone? Yes, Long?'

'Juvenal, Satire Eleven, sir.'

'You were fishing for the number, Long. It was Satire Ten. You can read it before we meet next Tuesday. Here—' Leasden threw a book to him – 'they do not make amusing criticism like that nowadays. One day, if you are clever, you will be able to write a satire of me.' *Goodness*, I thought, *it would be easier to walk to the moon.* Then I noticed Long's solemn look. He thought it was possible. 'Well, that is almost enough for a warm-up, except to ask you all to recite Cato the Elder's infamous quote.'

In unison we all said, '*Delenda est Carthago!*'

'Now a little tense testing for starters, before we do some unseens. Cooke, second person plural pluperfect indicative active of *parare.* Jones, the same for *habere,* and Long ditto for *sumere.* The rest of you write out the present subjunctive of *esse.* Ready, Cooke?'

'*Paraveratis*, sir.' Leasden nodded in acknowledgement of a correct answer.

Blow, I thought that answer was a million miles away from what I thought it would be. I was in the future perfect tense...

'Jones?'

'Ah...'

'Jones?'

'Ah... I – I thought it was *habueritis*.' (I wanted him to know I had used my brain). He seemed to divine this.

'Well. There is not a vacuum between your left and right auricle, I can see that, Jones! But I need the *pluperfect*, not the future. In this classroom we are not operating a time machine beloved of Americans. Have it ready by the time Long has answered. Long?'

'*Sumpseratis*, sir.' Long had answered far too quickly for me and I had never heard of *sumere* declining 'e' with a 'p' in it. Leasden turned slowly to me. I squeezed my legs together again.

'Jones?'

'Ahm, *habueras*, sir.' Leasden did not nod. I waited for the reprimand.

'Jones, if you were William Tell, you would have shot your son with your characteristic inaccuracy. *Habueras* is the singular of that tense. Now aim again, for with you it is *aiming,* not rock-like certainty – and try to hit the apple this time, and not the blessed boy.'

I thought quickly. '*Habueratis*, sir.'

There was a pause. Although he was short, Leasden appeared to me too tall and too close.

'The boy lives,' he said. He loomed over me, his nostrils flaring.

My contemporaries smirked quietly. I was impassive, I had learnt that any display of emotion cut no ice with Leasden. I looked out through the bay window. For me, Maths lessons in this room had an airy feel with light flooding in and ideas exchanged with freedom and delight. But here now I felt trapped. The Arcadian scenery outside mocked me as I squirmed and dodged Leasden's attack on my ignorance. He handed me another boy's attempts at the present subjunctive of *esse*.

'What do you think of that, Jones?'

I read it: *sim, sis, sit, simus, sitis, sint*. I couldn't improve on it.

'I think it is correct,' I replied.

'Yes, I thought you would say that. You don't *know* it is correct, do you?' He looked through the back of my head. I did not answer. At least I had learned not to hang myself. 'It *is* correct. Well, I am trying to help you pass, Jones. So you will carefully go through all their likely correct attempts. This will help you learn, and if they have any errors please inform me. While Jones does that, the rest of you look to page twenty-four. There you will find a piece of Xenophon. Please try and translate the first four sentences in your own time.'

I was the only one in the class who did not learn Greek. I looked through all the sheets. *Sim, sis, sit, simus, sitis, sint*. Then I came across one: *sim, sis, sHit, simus, sitis, sint*. I looked round the class. This was a set-up. The capital 'H' had been pencilled in by an unknown hand. If I said they were all correct and Leasden saw this, he could accuse me of putting in the capital 'H' or simply being complicit in an offence. All the others in the room ignored me. Either I would get done for sneaking on my fellow pupils or Leasden would maul me. Quickly I put the piece of paper in my mouth. Almost immediately Leasden moved.

'Jones, are they all correct? Can you hand them to me, please.'

'Er, yes, sir.' I handed them over to him.

'There appear to be only twenty one here, Brown. How do you account for that?' he asked, walking away from me. The class continued to hum as others busied themselves with Greek.

'I am not sure, sir.'

Leasden could see my real unease. His short, stocky body rotated on one point and across the classroom he faced me.

'Are you *eating*, Jones?'

Immediately there was a deadly hush; eating in class was a serious school offence. I froze.

'Spit the sweet or gum out, boy. I will not be responsible for you choking to death here. *Now!*'

I spat out the mangled paper. The whole place went theatrically quiet. Leasden moved forward in short brisk steps, took the piece of paper and opened it. His face went very dark. Everyone was expecting an inferno. He gave a grim smile and leaned down to me.

'"Greater love has no man than to die for his friends",' he quoted, *sotto voce*, while his shoulders sagged a little. He had visibly relaxed. No one in the class understood what was happening. 'See me after, Jones.' Leasden winked to me so no one could see. He then turned and faced the rest of the class.

'Someone else in this class is in very serious trouble, as you will all gather. It would be best if he stayed afterwards to ameliorate the wrath that is to come. I want you all to note that my previous sentence is a Delphic oracle style of quote. You are all – I emphasise *all* – to take note: someone else is guilty of a serious offence and should stay behind.'

I looked around at the others and tried to give a hint that I had no idea what was up.

'Now to some unseens from *Cook and Marchant,* page twenty-two at the top.'

We all grabbed our own copy of the blue textbook. 'Willoughby, you translate for us.'

Meum est propositum in taberna mori,
Ubi vina proxima morientis ori:
Tunc cantabunt laetius angelorum chori
"Sit Deus propitius huic potatori."'

Willoughby coughed and then in very serious and deliberate phrases spoke:

'It is my proposal to die in an inn
With a Christian my last glass shrinking
That angel choirs may sing as I am sinking
"God be merciful to his mode of thought."'

19

'Not bad, not bad at all. We can have a little humour with our unseen work, can't we? Now, Jones, the next on page twenty-two.'

"'Dic, canis, hic cuius tumulus?" "Canis." "At canis hic quis?"
"Diogenes." "Obiit?" "Non obiit sed abit."
"Diogenes, cui pera penus, cui dola sedes, ad manes abiit?" "Cerberus ire vetat." "Quonam igitur?" "Clari flagrat qua stella leonis, additus est iustae nunc canis ninc canis Erigonae."'

I could see at once that this was screamingly funny in Latin. Half the class was sniggering. Diogenes was always involved in humour and there was some sort of 'carry-on' about a dog's grave, Cerberus and a pun around *obiit* and *abit*. What it meant was quite beyond me. I had a stab at it. Without the opening cough beloved of the best classical scholars, I started my translation.

'Tell me, dog. This is whose grave? A dog. Whose dog? Diogenes'. Dead? Not dead, passed away. Diogenes who?' I paused. 'I am sorry, sir. I am stuck, sir.'

'I am sure you are.'

I saw Leasden bearing down on me. I jumped in terror.

'Oh-oh…' I looked up and saw the ceiling of my bedroom: at last I had escaped the dream. Through the bedroom windows I could make out the trees that shaded the railway station at Inverden. The dream had ended and I was back at home, safe in bed with an alert and awakened spouse.

'Where am I?'

'What's up?'

Next to me, my wife, Jill, looked at me in irritation. 'You have been moving and jumping around all night. No wonder I can't get to sleep for longer than twenty minutes. As for where you are – you are here; a vet in Scotland, Inverden. More importantly, where have you been with all this jumping around?'

'Bad dream,' I said. 'Belize and a lesson at school. A sort of nightmare.' I gulped for breath, relieved it was all over.

'Well, I think you are ridiculous. Belize was not such a bad place. Don't you remember, we often went out to the Cayes and snorkelled around all that coral? We slept out on the beaches of those islands with nothing but the stars and our sleeping bags. Why, I think you even went skinny-dipping with Eduardo in those forest streams high in the mountains. It really wasn't that bad at all.' A note of exasperation crept into her voice.

'Yes, yes, you're right,' I said not wanting an argument at midnight. 'There was definitely another side to it.' But she was not letting me get away with it completely.

'And a nightmare about a lesson. Haven't you grown up? How old are you?'

'Forty-something.' I couldn't do the Maths at midnight. '1957, hmm, forty-four.'

'Just – and you are still having bad dreams about school!' Jill's voice suddenly went all sweet and honey-like. 'Does Richard have baddy-baddy dreams about school? Do you want Mummy to write a note and take you out of school for a day? Get away from that nasty man? Perhaps have a word with the head and explain about my delicate little cherub...'

'Of course not!' I realised I probably deserved some mickey taking. 'I will be okay. It is just – well, he was a different kind of teacher. There was no one like him. He could engender real fear. His lessons were hell.' I raised myself on my elbows to make the point.

'Is that the one who sacked you from Greek?'

'The very one,' I sighed.

'Well, he seems to have had some common sense as far as I can see. Look at you and languages. You took French O level at two different boards in the hope if you failed one then you would pass the other.'

'I passed, both,' I rebutted, though I had to admit to myself that the substance of the accusation was true.

'Still, you are a duffer at languages. Whenever we have been in Europe I cringe when you open your mouth. Yes, science and vetting is your forte. He had some sense, that Latin teacher.'

'Latin and Greek,' I corrected her, 'that is the Classics.' But she had rolled over to sleep, thus indicating the conversation was over. Suddenly her head flipped back.

'What was he called?'

'Leasden,' I said. It was like mentioning a juju spirit.

'Leasden...' she repeated. 'Honest, forthright, hmm... yes. For once, a real man.' And she drifted off to sleep. I myself soon followed suit.

Unknown to me my encounters with Leasden had started.

Chapter Two

The critical period in matrimony is breakfast time.

AP Herbert.

The next morning I was in the downstairs bathroom when I heard the phone ring. Further down the corridor leading to the kitchen I heard Jill pick it up.

'Oh, hello,' she said in a lilting voice. The tone betrayed that it was someone she knew. I removed my head from the corridor and returned to my shaving. Three minutes later I wandered down the corridor past the pictures, some of which Jill had had mounted with brass lights above them. She liked that effect in this dark corridor.

'Well, I am sure you are looking forward to seeing him. He will be with you soon,' said Jill, smiling as I entered the kitchen. She immediately replaced the phone and picked up a piece of toast. She always had a light breakfast.

'Who was that?' I asked. It didn't quite ring true for a call of a farmer needing me out to see a beast.

'Oh, just your aunt.' She handed me a finger of toast with honey on it.

'Which one?'

'Aunt Sarah. Who else? Remember you are going down to spend the weekend with her. You promised ages ago you would visit. She was just checking that you were definitely coming.' Jill had turned round and was arranging her hair.

'Of course, I know that. But why didn't she want to speak to me? I thought I was her favourite nephew.' A note of irritation crept into my voice. I found myself a bowl of cereals.

'You are,' replied Jill tartly. She began moving round the kitchen, tidying bits and pieces. 'It is just as she said. She said you were always a little brief and short-tempered first thing, because she knew you had a lot on your mind about veterinary matters. So she just wanted to check with me. You know, most women can multitask.' She smiled. For me, it was bit early for this quick repartee.

'Fine, fine, okay. Anything else she said?'

'Oh, she wanted to remind you to bring everything. I said not to worry, as I would pack your case. You will have pyjamas, razor and so on. She also mentioned she had bumped into an old Chemistry or Latin teacher of yours at a bridge club. Can't remember his name.'

'Reid, Leasden, Smith, Robson?' There were so many teachers who came to mind.

'That is it. *Leasden*. Is that the one you mentioned last night?'

'Oh… well, I hope he is not around,' I observed tersely and uncharitably.

'It is odd, but your aunt seemed to know that and said he wouldn't be around. I wondered why she even bothered mentioning it.'

'Well, it was the event of that week – if not of the term,' I said.

'What?' said Jill, completely at a loss.

'Och, ne'er mind. Ken fit like.' Even I resorted to a form of the local dialect, Doric, when I was at a loss for words.

'Well, anyway I must go. Duty calls.' She smoothed down her black skirt, checked her black jacket, gave me a peck on the cheek, hopped over the dog and left by the back door. She paused for a second and assessed the path. Salt was liberally scattered across it, melting the ice; on either side of the path there was a couple of inches of snow. Taking the first few steps with care, she walked down the garden path with her nose slightly tilted up, as if to glean the best of the fresh morning air.

The modern Portia, I thought, about to outwit all who at law stand before her. God help them, I mused; for I wouldn't. As if on cue, two teenagers – Rachel and Edward – entered and started depositing all their schoolbags and other kit on the kitchen table. They then circumnavigated the kitchen, investigating all the kitchen unit surfaces for food, tea, cereals and money. They meandered round, picking up and putting down completely unrelated objects on the way.

'Yo, Dad! Mum away already?' asked one.

'Yes.' A slight sense of relief seemed to enter them. I was a soft touch, usually. Mum, in contrast, almost lined them up to attention before letting them on to school.

'She asked me to check that you, Edward, have your gym shoes. She didn't see them.'

'Deliberate error, bro?' cackled Rachel.

'Thanks for mentioning it, Dad.' Edward went into the cupboard and pulled them out.

After a few minutes I decided it was time we started the day. 'Okay – ready to go? I've got to get to work soon.'

'Sure, sure, Father.'

'"When shall we three meet again, in thunder, lightning or in rain?"'

'Dad, that is so uncool!'

'Yes, well past the sell-by date,' added the other.

'It is Shakespeare,' I defended myself. 'A rather obvious quote. He is great, you know.'

'Well, maybe, but I have him for English. Can I not have him for breakfast, please?'

'You guys have no sense of fun. You could at least try to reply with some humour.' I stood my ground.

'Oh, he wants humour at eight twenty,' observed one to another with eyes open wide. She then turned and shot at me, 'Not that you give Mum much humour at eight ten.'

'Rachel!'

'It's true, Edward. Anyway, here goes. Father, this is not your bard.' She took a deep breath.

'Go for it, Rach,' encouraged the other.

'"Oh Father, Father I would rather my bare bum appear
Than hear more hear more dull boring Shakespeare –
To moon in the gloom is not so rude
As to quote the bard when we're not in the mood."'

'Not bad,' I said.

'Yes, Father dear, and if you would give us time and money we would do it in time to rap music.' Rachel collected her assorted bags and files from the kitchen table.

'I think you had better get along.'

'Don't worry, Dad, we will meet again,' said Edward sympathetically.

'We'll meet again, we'll meet again – some day?' hummed Rachel as she exited with all her school gear.

'That is a little cruel,' said Edward, the more sensitive one.

'Come on, you lot. Best get out. Your dad can take that kind of thing. We all have got things to do.' They knew from my tone of voice I wasn't upset and so they hopped away up the road to school.

Twelve hours later we three did meet again – in the kitchen. All our respective work had been done long ago.

'I am going through to the sitting room to join Mum.' I checked that my mobile phone was charging. 'Any of you coming? There is supposed to be a Harrison Ford film on.' I braced myself for the jibes typical of the morning.

'Oh, yes!' said Edward. 'I haven't seen one of those for a while. Don't tell anyone, but they are as good as any video.' He barged his way past me toward the sitting room.

'Ya, Pop, I am coming to educate myself too. I will be along in a minute.' Rachel was writing in an exercise book on the kitchen table. I resisted my urge to tell her it was entertainment not education and followed Edward.

The fire gave a little burst of heat, the snow gusted and swirled against the sitting-room window. Each flake reflected briefly the blaze inside and then twisted back into the dark tinged with blue. Stretched across the red sitting-room carpet lay Maya. As a golden retriever she typified the warm colours of the room. Her coat, a mixture of pure gold and brassy coloured hairs, changed shades in time to the flames of the wood fire. The television flickered briefly as a particularly strong gust tugged at the aerial on the roof. The advertisements finished and the feature film, *Indiana Jones*, commenced. On the other side of the room, like Easter Island statues caught in the sunset, we three sat bolt upright on the sofa waiting for the entertainment to start. The door opened and closed quickly; we, the statuesque occupants of the sofa, remained immobile. Rachel sat cross-legged on the floor by Maya. She patted the dog and then set down her mobile phone on the deep carpet. I thought it was a scene of bourgeois domestic bliss. While I was sure the teenagers in the room would have felt a little uneasy about this description, they too enjoyed the moment.

'Oooh!' said one, as Indiana Jones started to jump from train carriage to train carriage.

'Great stunts,' murmured another appreciatively, as Indiana Jones leapt from the train onto a horse.

It was when Indiana Jones was wading through snakes that a phone rang.

'Rachel!' whispered Edward, implicitly accusing her of ruining the evening by allowing her teenage friends to barge in with what in normal circumstances would be a long phone conversation.

'No, not me,' was the curt reply from the daughter, her eyes still transfixed on the snakes, which were now mimicking spermatozoa by swimming around Indiana Jones's ankles in wave formation.

I looked at Jill in one of those knowing ways. The 'other' phone was passed to me. 'Inverden Vet Centre, can I help you?'

'Ah, is that Mr Jones, isn't it? I *am* glad *you* are on tonight.' (The caller had an unrealistically optimistic view of my talents.) 'It's Mr Smith from Hale here. I am sorry to call you late and at such a night like this. But I think I have a problem.' (Indiana Jones had just leapt onto a moving boat in the canals in Venice.) 'I just brought in a Highland cow from the field. What a job! She was not meant to be due for two or more months, but there is a string of stuff coming from the rear. What should I do?'

'Have you a halter and ropes?'

'Yes.'

'Well, I had better come down and see what's up.'

'Oh good, good, thank you.'

I put the phone down.

'Enjoy the film, I'm just going outside and may be some time.'

They hardly moved and had no doubt missed the Antarctic reference. The dog, a noted outdoor exercise fiend, wagged her tail but otherwise lay still as if to say 'see you later'. Indiana Jones was in mid air between a boat and dry land as I quit the cosy room.

My red Laguna wound its way through the piles of snow heaped up in a series of deposits lined at intervals along the small streets of our rural town. The ancient lantern-style street lights gave Inverden a rather twee, Dickensian veneer accentuated by the snow. You could easily imagine Scrooge suddenly popping round the corner, followed by a billowing cloud of snow, which would raise his frayed coat-tails.

Soon I was out on the main road. It was a wet dark path cutting through the unlit snowbound countryside. The snow, followed by hail, came down hard and buffeted the large front windscreen. 'Lord help,' I muttered. I knew the move from the sublime to the ridiculous to be very small for those in practice. Even with experience, I preferred the possibility of extra help in any form. After a few miles I found the turn-off and left the empty main road. No one with any sense was venturing out this night. This side road was a grey colour, and the slippery feel of the steering wheel and brittle noise from the tyres hinted at the danger on the surface. At the first right-hand corner the car started to go broadside. Avoiding the brake, I steered quickly into the skid, gave a squirt to the accelerator and straightened out. I could now clearly see the hard hailstones dancing on the road surface. They formed a carpet of ball bearings. The road stretched forward in an invitingly straight manner; there was little point in accelerating rapidly. A straight line successfully negotiated was an achievement. Three more curves, a rise and a dip, and I was at the end of the brief farm road. In traditional manner, all the farmhouse lights were on. I swung the car down the road, applied the brakes, skidded five yards and finished a yard or two from a set of gates. I got out and examined the skid: you could see in the slush the alternate tyre marks followed by skid marks indicating where the ABS system had applied and released itself.

In front of me, presenting her broadside from about fifteen yards distant, stood a Highland cow.

'Well there she is,' Mr Smith said, as though we were both admiring his new yacht safely deposited in the local marina. He had joined me beside the gate. A little string of white shiny material coming from her rear indicated that we would have to accomplish something tonight.

'We almost lost her, you know. The dog got out from the kitchen just as she was crossing the road up there.'

He indicated the road I had come along. I had visions of a calving Highlander running down the icy road chased by a dog until they both disappeared into the darkness of the mini-blizzard.

The cow was standing near a digger that had been used to muck out the open court on the right. The court was two-thirds empty but in the furthest third the muck was about five feet high above ground level. Mr Smith apologised for that, but he hadn't been expecting anything to calve for a while. A line of old tractors and gates prevented the cow escaping at the far end, while on the left an old stone farm building with troughs sealed off that side. A single powerful spotlight from this building illuminated the area.

'Well, we are going to have to get her by her horns and then tie her to one of the court stanchions, okay?'

All agreed. So, over the gate, farmer, wife, his son and I went. It took us over half an hour to get a rope around the two horns. The cow wasn't aggressive, which was a relief, but she was by no means cooperative. I could not get near her, so the family – who knew her well – tried, with more success. First she tried to burrow her way through the line of tractors and gates. She found an opening a normal cow would have got through but due to the size of her horns she was unsuccessful. When she reversed out of that we managed to get a loop around just one horn. The distance between the two points was surprisingly large; three of us had ropes. Due to the wide horns she couldn't even get herself into the crush. It was standing by for some reason. She climbed up the unmucked part of the court; since she usually gave me a wide berth I volunteered to climb up the slope with its uncertain footing, hoping she wouldn't have a go. Down she came and headed for the gates. We all knew she could leap those easily if so minded, and immediately ran to head her off. From then on one person stood guard at the gates. Just as Mrs Smith was succeeding in getting a rope on the cow she flicked her horns and caught Mrs Smith on the cheek.

We all stopped. Fortunately, no damage was done. The cow hid in the shadow created by the digger. Eventually the weird pantomime finished when we managed to get one rope round the base of both her horns. We pulled her towards the stanchion, trying to keep the stanchion between us and her in case she came forward suddenly. When she was about two feet away we put a second rope on her and set her at that distance. Any closer and we risked locking her to the stanchion. This would be a problem if she bent her neck while leaping: when she came down she could break it.

'Well, that is two stages accomplished. Getting her in from the field, and getting her tied up,' I said. 'Now the moment of truth.'

I put my hand inside and found two large feet, and a little further back a head but no sign of life.

'She is calving. We will have to use the machine.'

I didn't mention the fact that the feet appeared large, the sidewalls of the hips appeared a little tight and there was an annoying bump protruding up from the ventral floor where the pubic symphysis occurred.

'I didn't mention this, Mr Jones. A week after I purchased her the seller told me she had a dead calf last year. So although she is nearly six she still has not had a live calf,' Mr Smith informed me.

I thought ruefully how many dairy cows would be almost completing their careers at that age, and here was a Highlander trying to start her breeding life. The last thing I wanted was a Caesar in these circumstances.

'Do you have a little water for me to wet the calving ropes?' I asked.

Mr Smith tried to switch on the tap by the trough but it was frozen solid. I dipped the rope in the glacial trough water and then started a typical *pas de deux* with the cow. She stood for the first rope but twisted around a lot for the second. With the possibility of a Caesar looming I wasn't going to sedate her at this stage. We applied the calving aid. At the first pressure the cow reacted strongly, jumping everywhere. This had an added adventure because the calving aid now created a six-foot metal lever stuck to her backside. She became remarkably able at swinging it round: we ducked and weaved to avoid it. Finally she settled down and we put on more pressure. Unfortunately, the feet would come but not the head: it was not engaging. Boy, I thought, This really could be a Caesar...

Still, I decided to put on a head rope and was glad I had not roped her down as the head ropes procedure is much easier when the cow is standing. While I grunted and sweated putting on the rope, Mrs Smith stroked the cow's back and talked to her the way females talk about childbirth. This may seem silly to an outsider, but it can on occasion settle the cow a little.

Head rope on, and we started all over again. Mrs Smith pulled on the rope and managed to successfully engage the head into the pelvis. The feet, with the calving aid's assistance, came next. At that juncture the cow toppled over and landed with a thud on her side and settled in a two-inch-deep mud slurry. It always fascinates me how at that particular point if a cow falls over it is in one single smooth motion with both hind legs parallel. The move is not graceful, but would appeal to the aesthetic tastes of a lumberjack. There was no time to dwell on this. We quickly adjusted the ropes and re-engaged the calving aid; we knew we were fully committed and so just 'went for it'.

The head soon popped out. I instructed Mrs Smith to loosen the head rope while the others maintained all the correct angles and pressures. The chest came, followed by hips and with a final 'sploosh' the hind legs. It had been a stiff but reasonable pull. The calf gave a cough. It was alive. We then resembled a gun crew at the Earl's Court Tournament. Acting with alacrity and moving as one man, the three of us dragged and lifted the calf over the uncertain terrain to the gate twelve yards away. We quickly raised the hind legs over the top bar and 'hung' the calf there. I scuttled away to the empty trough for my gear and the Dopram. By the time I came back he was blinking and breathing a bit. I squirted half a cc up the nose and injected him with one cc into the muscle. We examined him. It was a bull calf. Dad was judged to be a Shorthorn. With every moment he seemed to be looking brighter. Mr Smith's son went to the middle of the covered court and made an apron of fresh straw. The 'guncrew' whisked the calf to his new accommodation free from hail and snow. His navel was dipped with iodine.

We turned to look at the dam. All we could see was steam rising from a mound of animated being covered with long red hair, one horn sticking out like a forlorn radar cone, a long silvery metal bar sticking out from one side. All this was surrounded by dark mud and highlighted by a strong spotlight. You could be forgiven for thinking that this was a scene from an American *Close Encounters*-style sci-fi movie. Occasionally a whoosh of misty smoke would come from amid the hair to confirm that the alien was alive.

'Well, I had better do my checks,' I said. I bent down at the rear and confirmed the absence of a twin. While I gave a prophylatic injection in the rear plate, I noticed that the cow didn't flinch when Mrs Smith cleaned the udder with the coldest water imaginable. That concerned me. I elected to put a bottle of calcium under the skin. The risk–benefit ratio of one in the vein didn't justify it from my viewpoint; besides, it would take five minutes to clip the hair around the neck to find the skin. All done and with straw under the udder, we debated how to release her. A significant number of recently calved Highlanders are extremely dangerous for a few days post-partem: they are hypersensitive to the possibility that you may have 'plans' for their calf. Thus they will quite simply seek to destroy you.

We agreed a plan to release the ropes and flee for the gate. Once we arrived at the gate we found she hadn't moved bar raising her head. We then in turns volunteered to simulate 'bait' by going close to her to see if she would rise to engage in the chase. Still no joy. We then examined her more closely. In my mind I could divide her into three sections. The front third was bright, alert and angry. When we encouraged her to rise the head flicked this way and that trying to catch us with her horns. She would stick her tongue out and give the best a bovine can do for a mean hiss – 'Hhuurrgh' – and the tongue would remain stuck out, trembling with frustration and anger. The middle third of the body was calm and composed, with normal breathing and rumination. The last third appeared lifeless. Try as we might she wouldn't rise. So we then rolled her off her left hind leg onto her right. Up she got in a flash and almost as quickly we reached the gate.

We turned round, breathless, but on the safe side of the gate. She had made a beeline for her first living calf and was busy licking it. We could hear all the right noises coming from mum and offspring. We retired to the farmhouse where the Smiths enthusiastically helped me clean all my gear. They were happy;

earlier in the day they had faced the very real possibility of an aborting cow in the middle of severe weather and now, by good fortune, they had a cow with a living bull calf safe and well. Mrs Smith pushed a bar of chocolate into my fist while I made my apologies for a quick return to my duty.

I returned down the empty wintery road. At the kitchen door I let myself in. A single soft light was left on. All was quiet. The *Indiana Jones* adventurers had gone to bed, no doubt satiated with their vicarious thrills. The cat looked down on me from the top of a kitchen unit. She fixed me with an owl-like stare, blinked twice, yawned and then fixed her gaze on a point behind and to the left of me. She had seen it all before. I sat down and enjoyed the silence. That had been a little adventure. Admittedly, it had been encapsulated within the bounds of farms, yet it had been real and not celluloid. Thankfully, not every night was like that, I mulled. That brought back memories of other vets. Malcolm, my first boss, who confided to me one morning how he had found himself in a fix the night before. At two a.m. he was in a small copse of saplings trying with two farm hands to secure a calving dairy heifer. Unfortunately she had six equally excited heifers for company. The rain was bucketing down and the ground was slippery. They had been charging around the copse for three quarters of an hour trying to catch the heifer and dodge her mates, who were crashing through the small wood. The saplings were always impeding the ropes. Now, five hundred kilos plus of maiden heifer at speed in the dark is a dangerous proposition.

'Do you know, Richard, when I thought of you and all the others tucked up and cosy I said to myself, "This is madness. I am well off and too old to need this kind of crazy game!" But you know one other thing? I wouldn't have wanted to be anywhere else in the world. Strange, isn't it?'

Malcolm calved his heifer. I reasoned that for many of us there would often be a little magic in the midnight madness of farm practice. I had a glass of milk and went to bed.

Chapter Three

Pressure, under pressure.

Queen

The next day I went in to the practice and found Neil, my partner, already in before me. He had his white lab coat on and was methodically working his way through a procedure on the lab bench surface.

'Morning, Neil,' I greeted him.

'Oh, morning Richard. Busy night? You look a little unkempt.'

'Oh,' I replied, nonplussed. Most mornings, my style of dress left a space for improvement. Usually, before the first consultation, acting on advice of the girls, I straightened myself up. Once famously I had stymied their attempts to check my appearance by turning up with two ties on. They had not been sure I was with it; I had reassured them that if they gave me a cup of tea I would be fine.

'Well, given your baseline of dress—' here he emphasised the word 'base'— 'you are a little below par.' Neil was a keen golfer.

'Well, I feel okay, thanks. Just a little tired. The night before I had insomnia; a nightmare, in fact. I don't usually get those. Then last night I was out late at Smith, Hale. Calving a Highlander.'

'Get on fine?'

'Yes, I was lucky. It all worked out.' I watched Neil move along the bench with his back to me. We knew each other well enough to speak with our backs to each other. On occasion we had had to operate on either side of an animal unable to see each other at all.

My partner in the practice was about ten years older than me. He was the original unreconstructed male. Born in an age where a man was a man and women had women's work to do, he occasionally appeared unforgiving in his attitude to the world. But when he was a young lad his dad, the local vet for Inverden, had often castrated as many as thirty horses in one morning. The horses had been well held, twitched, and the vet had taken a calculated risk. So it was that Gordon believed in the ancient codes of chivalry, honour and commitment. He would rise to his feet if a woman entered the room and open doors for them. There were some things he did not expect women to do, and in his perfect world there were clubs were men preferred the company of other men – not for some strange sexual fling but for the enjoyment of deep and trusted fellowship where matters which could not be mentioned in front of ladies were spoken of.

This did not mean that you could pass him off as predictable, he was too intelligent for that. He had been Head of School on merit. He admired the pursuit of excellence. In his eyes the sexes were possible spiritual equals, but they were not physically or mentally the same. Thus there were some jobs that men were better at than women and vice versa. The farmers he served were demanding folk whose compliment for a brilliant piece of work was 'nae bad'. In these circumstances you placed your most excellent workers up against the type of task they were best suited to. The world did not allow for second bests in planning for success. It was admitted that in the outcome there was still a role for time and chance. Nevertheless, every day on the farms nature told him that the sexes were different in their abilities, and this he applied in his own approach to life. The adjectives and adverbs I used when I thought of him were committed, courageous, alacrity, occasionally tempestuous and, when the mood suited him, courteously charming. He always lived life to the full. There was a famous occasion when he had been called to the mart to stitch up a stirk that had severely lacerated itself. Halfway through the suturing the sedated and comatose animal had quite unexpectedly delivered a ferocious kick. The kick hit Neil, who was bent down at the stirk's rear. The foot caught his head. Neil was knocked unconscious for about twenty seconds. Undeterred, and ignoring the pleas of the workers to go to hospital for a check, Neil brushed them aside, re-addressed the wound, and finished the stitching up. No beast was going to get the better of him, accident or no.

His speed in all areas of life was renowned. Some farmers

nicknamed him 'Blink and he's gone'. Not surprisingly, he was a keen downhill skier. Neil was determined that 'age should not wither him': early morning he could be found swimming a considerable number of lengths in the local pool, yet he was over fifty. He could, when he stood still, get on with anyone. As a local lad, he could speak Doric perfectly; he could also speak with a pure English accent which would not betray his Scottish roots, and was passable at German and French. Although he was not too keen on heart-to-heart talks, and the feeling was mutual, when we did talk about the hard things of life I always found him amazingly charitable and understanding. Such was my partner.

'Well, I was hoping you would do Duncan's test...' From his tone of voice I could see he was worried that I would say I was not up for it. 'You could leave early then, as it is your weekend off. Get your weekend off to an early start Friday afternoon.' That was the bait.

'Sure, fine. Besides, I tested the first half of the herd earlier in the week. It went quite smoothly. We were finished within a couple of hours.'

'Precisely, and anyhow he's hinted he wants you to go. It will keep some consistency to all the paperwork. Movement books and so on.' I knew that that mattered little but let it pass. 'Ten o'clock start. I said you would be there.'

Neil still presented his back to me while his voice hinted a little humour: he loved it when his plans fell into place. As if remembering some manners he turned and changed the subject. 'Up to anything special this weekend?' Unlike him, I couldn't boast a quick jaunt to Madrid, Paris or Dublin. Neil loved to rush away for a city break and see something interesting.

'Well, I am going down to Norbury to see my aunt,' I informed him.

'Norbury, Norbury...' Neil fished.

'I was at school there, Neil. Norbury College.' Neil's head nodded in recollection. 'There is a grammar school in the town as well,' I added.

'Quite, quite.' Neil couldn't resist a slightly turned-up lip at my ingrained snobbery. But he also did not know if I had raised it as bait for him to nibble at. We often kidded each other.

'My aunt used to invite me out for Sunday lunch at least twice a term. She demanded I bring friends, probably to see if I had any. I now think it was also to see what company I kept, and so report back to my parents, who were abroad. She was always very generous but never poked her nose into internal school matters.'

'Aunts can either be awful or very sensible, can't they?'

'Well, she was up to scratch. She even used to ply us with drink and stuff us full of food, saying it would keep us going until the next time. Anyway, I became quite attached to her. I did not fully realise the implications at the time but her husband died a year or two before I went to Norbury. She was left bringing up two children. They have done well.'

'Quite a character, your aunt, then,' observed Neil as he played with some test tubes.

'Yes, but you wouldn't think so. She is a little like Miss Marple. Well, not so quaint, but there is much more to her than you would think in conversation.' Neil smiled and left the room. I began searching around for the kit to do the blood tests. Soon I had collected all the equipment: a halter; a hundred empty vacutainer blood tubes; a hundred needles; two needle holders; numbered labels for each tube; a recording book; two pens; and a quantity of paper towels.

I walked back into the office to find the two receptionists, Emma and June, busy preparing for the day's work. We called them 'girls', which belied their considerable talents. Both could have easily completed university degree courses, but for various reasons they left studying early. Neil and I suspected one of them, Emma, possessed the highest IQ of anyone in the pactice. This we deduced from, among other evidence, her 'O' level results, which were better than ours, and the lightning speed with which she completed any accounting task. The girls solved matters in refreshing, novel ways since they possessed intelligence but had never been moulded by any academic minds. Neil avoided any attempt to dictate to them and often whispered to me, 'Let them have their head: it is much better.'

'Is there anything you want me to take to Duncan's farm?' I asked June.

'Yes, could you take these replacement tags?' She handed me a padded envelope. Inside the envelope were a set of large yellow tags with an exceedingly complex series of numbers. This set of numbers would tally with the 'passport' the farmer held in Duncan's office. He would have a box full of 'passports' – one for every individual animal he had. If any died or left the farm then the passport had either to be handed in, with an explanation, or passed on to the new owner. The administrative system was gargantuan. Few in the general public had any idea about it. We knew more about the whereabouts of our cattle than the police did about any old lags who had been let out...

'Oh yes, could you also take two five dose bottles of calf pneumonia vaccine? Wait, I will get them from the fridge.'

Emma went next door and came back with a cool bag with the vaccine inside. I looked inside and checked the numbers of vials. This was no insult to them. It was always worth double-checking. I had a theory that when it came to complex administrative actions with, for example, reading tag numbers, one should expect an error rate of one in thirty tags being either read or written down incorrectly.

'Does he need any more needles and syringes, do you know?' I asked.

'No, he told me he was fine. He had just got his numbers a little wrong and dropped a bottle.'

'Richard, before you go do you mind seeing Mrs Little? Her cat needs a booster. The others are busy.' Emma began to organise me.

'Sure.' I smelt a hint of a joke. Sure enough, when I turned into the waiting room and announced Mrs Little, I found myself confronted by an enormous bathtub of a lady. Out of the corner of my eye I saw Emma and June holding their hands together as if in prayer. They were watching me closely to see if I betrayed any emotion. I looked at them directly as if to say, 'I know what you two are up to.' Meanwhile, Mrs Little was having difficulty with her cat cage. The cage was attached to her corpulent shape and stuck out at right angles from her. This was an elevation the cat objected to.

'Here, let me take that, please.' I quickly moved forward, grabbed the cage and ushered her into the consulting room. Her breaths could be clearly heard as she stood, statuesque, in the centre of the room. The cat cage, which had a label tied to it, mimicked an exhibit in a criminal case. For a second I wondered what on earth a surgeon would do if he ever had to operate on Mrs Little's body. Get a power saw? I kicked myself. I had a job to do, and besides, it was unkind. She could, after all, be a generous old soul.

'Oh, I know what you are thinking,' she said.

'Really?' I said, worried.

'Yes, you will be giving me a row for not bringing Rambo back in time. I know he is overdue his booster vaccination. Here is his card and the reminder your nice girls sent me.'

Relieved, I looked at the card. Rambo had only missed his booster by two weeks: on occasion I encountered people who had forgotten to bring the animal in for two years.

'He won't need to start the whole course again, will he? That might be a bit more than I could afford.' Mrs Little looked at me with hope. 'I know that you are supposed to do the best for them, and I try. Worm him four times a year, like.' She took another deep, whistling breath.

'Don't worry, Mrs Little. I can see from here that you look after him well.' I neglected to say that I had been surprised at the great weight of the cage. 'He will be fine with just one injection. It is the one with flu and leukaemia, isn't it?' I queried. If money was tight I wanted to be sure that she knew what was happening. Some people who really were broke could only afford an injection against cat flu and parvovirus. They couldn't afford the additional cover for feline leukaemia. We did not like this approach, but recognised that some vaccine given was better than none.

'Oh, yes, that is the one I saved up for,' she said enthusiastically. 'Your nice lady vet got me to have Rambo done for leukaemia two years ago. It is on the card.'

'I see that,' I acknowledged. Opening the top of the cage, I admired a magnificent specimen. I pulled him out and put him on the table. He was, I estimated, seven kilos of pure athleticism.

'That is all muscle!' I looked at him in awe. 'I bet he kills everything in sight.'

'Oh, yes he is real killer and – so fit,' enthused Mrs Little her eyes brightening up. 'Not like me at all. But then I have hormones to blame for my weight – almost nothing I can do short of a cork at each end. Even the doctors are giving up on me.' She was staring at Rambo and had also let her thoughts wander. 'Oh, I shouldn't have said that!' She looked up guiltily. Her face went pink and a little bead of perspiration appeared.

'Don't worry, I heard nothing and forget immediately, Mrs Little. Let me see this athlete again.' And I began to clinically examine him. He let me handle him. Apart from one chipped upper canine he seemed in the pink of health. All the time Rambo stared ahead, pretending to ignore all my prodding and poking. I loaded my syringe and injected him in the scruff. Rambo blinked slowly.

'Laid-back kind of character, isn't he?'

'Oh yes, until he sees something he wants to catch – then he's a different beast altogether!' replied Mrs Little.

I handed her the completed vaccination card. 'Do you need any worming pills for him?'

'No, I am fine, thank you. I got some last week.'

'I will take the cage out for you,' I suggested.

'That is fine, if you could. My husband is in the Ford Focus. I'll go and pay.' She passed through in front of me. When I returned to the office I found June and Emma looking at me.

'Ha ha,' I said. 'She's a very nice lady.'

'What's this?' Neil came in, clutching some medical history cards.

'Oh, the girls were just trying me on sending me out to an enormous Mrs Little.'

Neil listened, paused and added, 'Yes, I think they tried something similar on me. Didn't work, of course.'

I turned to the girls. 'Explain.'

'Well, it is like this,' said one, 'a new client came.'

'Clients,' added the other.

'And you know how we like to do the best for them.'

'Go on,' I was not catching the drift at all.

'One of the two...' said Emma.

'...gentlemen,' said June, raising one eyebrow.

'...asked to see a male vet.'

'That was not his exact phrase. He said his dog Rex needed to be seen by "an unambiguous man". Rex, you see, doesn't get on with women.'

'And let me guess, girls. Rex is an Alsatian?'

'Yes, and he certainly doesn't like women. When I put my head out of the reception window he came for me,' said Emma, damning the dog in one phrase.

Neil was sitting down tapping the medical cards on the desk as he listened to this explanation. He interjected, 'There are two men in the practice. Why did you chose me?'

'Ah, Mr Morrison, we all know you are a real man, definitely an unambiguous man. No, seriously, that is meant to be a compliment!' They could see both of us moving in our seats. 'No offence, Richard, but you are softer, more artistic and so on.'

'Neil goes to art galleries too!'

'Aha!' Neil exclaimed. 'But perhaps they knew you had been a naval cadet in an English public school. Thus an element of doubt crept into their minds regarding you as a choice. And so our two ladies acted as judge and jury and preceded to set me up.' Neil pointed his medical cards at me and then tapped them twice with some force.

'So what happened?' I was interested.

'Unbeknownst to me, I end up in the room with a couple of rampant gays,' said Neil.

'Neil, *really*…' I cautioned him. 'We are supposed to be broad-minded now in the twenty-first century; and anyhow, how did you know?'

'It was obvious,' said June. 'I have worked behind a bar for so long I can spot them. Addicts, cross-dressers, gays: I know them all. Most I can spot before the drink makes them tell me. You would be surprised at the number of transvestites even up here in the Highlands. Why, last Saturday one even told me he had an evening dress just like mine back at home.'

'Yes,' said Neil. 'I suppose it was not that they were gay that knocked me off my stride. The body language was obvious. Mind you, they were standing, Richard, closer than you or I are ever to our wives in public. In fact, it was the condition of the dog that finished me. It had anal furunculosis. Did you know that, girls?'

'We did,' they chanted like little girls from *The Mikado*.

'Was it bad, oozing and all that?' I enquired.

'Yes, it was unpleasant and sore all around the anus. All the poor dog could do was bite and lick at its rear end. That just made it worse,' Neil explained.

'Sounds nasty. Perhaps we could sort it with some cryo if it doesn't come right soon?' I suggested.

'Agreed; so I had to explain to those two how the condition around the anus was made worse by tight, damp humid conditions. They both had incredibly tight jeans, just like Nureyev! Then I had to explain how trauma in that area – even minor trauma – could make it much worse. I mentioned it was often found in that breed. This phrase kept on popping in to my head and I had to resist saying it... *As you no doubt will well know, bodily hygiene in that area is crucial to a satisfactory lifestyle.* In the end I just spoke in short monosyllabic sentences, I was so scared I would cause offence.' Thus Neil pleaded his defence.

'Yes, they were impressed with that,' noted June.

'They said they like your simple approach. Wondered if you had been a bereavement counsellor,' concurred Emma.

'There, Neil. Shows you can be quite a star. New client well pleased,' I said.

The girls giggled.

'Yes, that reminds me, Mr Morrison,' added June enthusiastically, 'that was their parting shot. They said Neil had satisfied them so well they would recommend him to all their friends.' At this, Neil looked stunned.

'So you satisfied them, Neil. Satisfied their desires. Fine by me... You just do your straight vet job as well as you did there, and everyone's a winner. Perhaps we'll all learn more this way.'

'Who's next to see?' Neil asked, changing the subject abruptly.

'Mr Kiwatowski for you,' said June handing him the card.

Neil didn't blink. The Kiwatowskis had come to Inverden during the war. There were quite a few now to be found amongst all the traditional Scottish surnames like Gordon, Whyte, Morrison, Irvine MacDonald and so on.

'It's time I went off to Duncan's test. Okay by you?' I asked.

'Yes, fine, see you later.' The girls were more or less in control of the day-to-day running. They directed who went where for emergencies and new calls.

I drove out of the town past a garden centre identified by three flag-posts carrying tattered flags of St Andrew, St George and the Union. The wind had damaged them. There was a roundabout when I came up to the main north-south road. I crossed over it and headed down a long valley bordered by hills. In the distance out at the far end of the valley one or two distant blue peaks of the Grampian Mountains could be made out. After I had been through a small town I turned right away from the Grampians and up into the hills. Old barbed-wire fences or low stone dykes demarcated the fields on either side. Most of the land was limited for use in cattle, sheep or barley. One pasture had a series of standing stones in it; they had odd ancient Celtic writings or pictures on them that an expert could make out.

Duncan's farm was high up one of these hills. At that altitude it was eligible for hill farmer subsidy. It also opened it up to the possibility of appalling weather conditions. The hills around the farm were beautiful. Majestic was not an excessive compliment to them. However, the showers of rain, hail, sleet and snow that came down off them required a bitter display of strength from any mammal that was to survive there.

When I arrived the wind was gusting and the rain was on the point of turning to hail. The characteristic quiet solitude of the hills was completely absent. The mild din I met was caused by the combination of vocal cattle unhappy at being moved about, the whining of the wind, the trees creaking, and the rattles and rumbles of the farm building weathering the storm. Shallow puddles rippled as the wind tried to lift up the surface water. Occasionally it would succeed and a little spray would whip off the puddles. I positioned my car in one of the few dry spots on the farm, close to a big sliding door.

I put my head in and surveyed the situation; it was a little quieter inside. Duncan, his brother Iain and two other helpers were obviously busy making preparations, setting up gates, checking vaccines, tags, checking the crush, placing feed in troughs. It was a large, tall, sprawling building not unlike an amalgamation of three or possibly four ancient warehouses. All seemed to be going to plan. I brought in my blood-collecting materials and closed the door behind me. It all became cosier now and a little quieter. There was one large group of cows kept just outside the building. They were penned in and had a plentiful supply of silage in mobile troughs beside them. I noticed that they were hammering in to the feed. On a cold day like this most cows would eat well. The subsequent heat generated from the breakdown of the grass in their rumen fermentation chambers would buffer them against extremes of temperature. A man could probably not cope with these weather changes; however, I did know that one of the warmest places to be in a cold day such as this was with one arm deep inside the backside of a cow checking her for pregnancy. Fortunately, Duncan was not offering me that job today.

'Are you ready?' he said

'As I ever could be,' I replied.

'Well, I hope it goes as well as last time. These ones seem a bit jittery today,' he commented. 'My brother and the others are handling them as quietly as possible.'

He had divined my main concern. If the cows were roughly handled they would play up even more and our job could be made twice as hard. Duncan and I stood on a pass about fifty metres long and three metres wide which stretched across the width of these conjoined buildings. To the left of the pass there was a drop of a few feet. This left side area contained a large number of fattening (store) animals about twelve to eighteen months old. As these young stock were not significant to Brucellosis[1] they would not be blood sampled. The cows entered the pass from an opening on the right about fifteen metres away from us. A gate stopped them turning right and the high barriers which kept in the store beasts helped guide the cows to the left and down towards us.

A few yards short of us, two gates would angle in towards the right, starting from the rail. This would guide the cows into the crush and create a space to the left of it for us to work in. A spare gate would be moved behind the cow as she entered the crush; it could be used to squeeze her in if necessary. The crush was bolted to the floor and side wall to restrain it. Unrestrained, it was

---

[1] Brucellosis is mainly found in adult breeding stock, where it causes abortion outbreaks. The disease, if transmitted to man, is quite severe and long lasting and is commonly called undulant fever.

possible for a very fractious cow to rock it so severely that it might fall on one side. At the very least, a crush needed to be stabilised by a gate attached to the end as a crude form of anchor. The essence of a crush was to be an oblong box about the size relevant for a large cow, with a gate at the rear and a method of restraining the head at the front. They varied enormously in their efficiency and design. As I examined the various barriers and restraints I came to the conclusion that we were about to use a well-designed set-up. What the cows did to it in the next few hours surprised me.

The first cow erupted from the byre onto the pass. She immediately turned left, saw us and paused for a second. Then she purposefully headed for the crush and slammed into the front of it. She seemed intent in getting the examination over with quickly. As we were about to put a halter on her head she reversed back in one swift motion and delivered herself a terrific crack to the back of her skull against the restraint. This collision between skull and metal would have knocked any one of us out: the noise resounded through the building. However, all cattle have an extra layer of bone with an air pocket surrounding the skull bones which are immediately protecting the brain. This amounts to a very strong crash helmet: I have only once seen a man knock a cow out with a blow; this so terrified me that I disappeared until the man had cooled down.

Duncan carefully put on the halter to the unaffected cow and pulled her head up and to the right. This presented the side of the neck to me for blood sampling from the jugular vein. The cow continued to bang her head against the crush. We paused a little, and once she was still I took the blood sample. We opened the crush door and stood to one side as the cow leapt out in an overweight bovine parody of a delicate skip by Bambi. The beef cow had a solid build with stocky short legs typical of a suckler cow. Her large backside would have graced a rugby pitch better than a ballet. All of Duncan's beasts would be a variation on this theme, and a mixture of beef breeds: Aberdeen Angus; Beef Shorthorn; Charolais; Simmental; and Limousin. Duncan looked at me and then at his disappearing beef cow. He briefly raised his eyebrows.

The next cow came in quietly and just stood there. When I tried to raise the vein to find the blood vessel, to my surprise there was hardly anything to see.

'Well, she either has no blood or is so cold that none is circulating very well,' I commented. Duncan saw my predicament. Eventually, knowing more or less where the blood vessel should be, I just stabbed at it. I missed twice and wasted two blood tubes, which is all I would normally waste for a whole test. Now I had done it on the second cow. The third tube filled with blood. I turned to my box and placed the correct label onto the tube while Duncan let the cow go.

The third cow came in and poked her head through the crush correctly, but then started a weaving motion with her head which made it very difficult for Duncan to put on her halter. Eventually he got it on and had more or less restrained her. I was just about to push the needle in to collect the blood when she suddenly twisted and moved her head. This neat move spun the needle back on me and stuck the needle into the tip of my thumb. It was quite painful and blood appeared at a rate, covering the outside of the tube. I quickly carried on and took the blood sample.

'I think we might be in for a rough ride,' I commented to Duncan.

'They're not so well behaved as the ones before,' he said in a deadpan manner.

'It may be that with the sudden cold weather the blood magnesium level has gone down. They can get very irritable then. Though they may not take staggers, they are a problem to handle. We'll see.'

'Yes,' said Duncan, 'maybe.'

I could be loquacious as any Englishman. Equally well, Duncan could be as brief and to the point as any Scot; we understood each other. The next few cows were just as tricky as the others to handle, but with our experience we managed. Then I found that the blood tubes were getting covered liberally with blood from my thumb. So I found some spare tube labels marked X202 171, X202 172 and X202 173. These three very sticky labels bandaged my thumb and formed a *petite tourniquet*. We were just beginning to get into our stride with a fluency and rhythm when the cows found a new trick. Three of a group of ten cows managed to hit the front of the crush with such force that the vibration opened the front door. They then careered away beyond us, banging against the side walls like a lorry out of control, unsampled. Each time we ignored this. Instead, we blood sampled another couple of cows and then went on to the byre to look for the unsampled ones. By then they would have calmed down a fraction. Very efficiently, we led them back to the group of untested cows. By the third cow everyone stopped. Duncan's brother, Iain, was not keen on sending cattle up for us to test if we were losing them.

A careful examination was made of the locks and snibs of the crush. Duncan was a little embarrassed because he had checked them out the day before and they had appeared fine. Someone spotted a piece of metal which was stopping a latch from descending correctly. This caused men to disperse and look for extension leads, torches and a metal grinder to perform a running repair. Sparks flew everywhere and the blood test looked more like a garage than an animal handling facility.

By this time the cows were becoming even more restless. We had had the well-behaved ones first and the minor deviants were now beginning to appear. A cow instead of turning down to our crush decided to go straight ahead and jump over the gates and join the feeding beasts. In the process she entangled both her hind feet in the gate and pitched forward. She ended up with her neck hanging down to the feeding beasts and her feet anchored by the crushed gate. Her rear remained attached to the pass and the gate. She had the wisdom to cease struggling and just lay there. Duncan observed that at least I had an immobile cow; 'perhaps I could blood sample her?' Since her head was low down, all the blood had gone to the head, and while someone steadied her I took blood from the neck. The tube filled instantly. We still did not know what to do with her. She seemed to have quietened down, so three of us lifted her back up to the pass but she was still stuck with her feet entangled in the gate, which by now was a parody of its original shape. The consensus was to leave her alone. It was judged she would be better by herself in getting out of the predicament. So we found a replacement gate to stop cows leaping in to the feeding beasts and left her there. Duncan's brother and his helpers went off to find us some more beasts to test. This was the right decision. Five minutes later there was a terrible noise of iron bouncing against concrete as the cow got up and shook the gate off her feet. She walked away, apparently unharmed.

The bull came and went with no ceremony. I took blood from his tail vein. Paradoxically, he was docile. It is often that way; when you expect trouble from a bull it is easy. On other days if one is a little casual in approach they can suddenly turn out to be extremely dangerous.

By now we were coming up to the fortieth cow, there being over sixty to test. A cow entered the crush but failed to put her head through the opening at the end. She was impossible to sample without her head being restrained, and she appeared to be aware of this. Instead she put her head high up in the air and started sniffing around. We would do the same if, say, we thought something was burning. This was a warning sign to us. The cow was looking for somewhere to jump. We knocked her head down but she avoided our hands and kept her nose pointed to the heavens. Duncan turned around for the halter to place on her head, and in that moment she leaned back and reared up on her hind feet.

'Watch out,' I stated calmly. By now I was picking up Duncan's habits of understatement. She was obviously trying to jump sideways out of the crush and might land on top of us. Fortunately, she aimed her leap for the far side of the crush away from us. However she was only able to get half her body out. She vainly kicked with her hind feet but they hardly touched the floor of the crush. She was straddled six feet up, half in half out of a crush and on top of a wall. Duncan, unruffled as ever, advised me to take blood from her tail. She was presenting her tail straight out of our side of the crush halfway along its length. His was sound advice, so I soon had the blood sample, but this left us with the immediate problem: how to get the cow out of the crush. To my horror I remembered that the side on which she was attempting to leave had a drop of fifteen feet or more on the other side. This also meant we had no purchase on that far side to push her back. If we went to that side, she would be high above us. Duncan could not get a tractor in there.

The cow by now was getting breathless: the wall she was

stranded on was compressing her sternum and the whole of her chest. We put a rope around her neck and tried to pull her back on to our side but it was hopeless. With the cow by now being in some distress, we had no option but to try and lift her over the side of the crush and down a sizeable drop. Duncan and the others slowly raised and pushed her hips up and over the wall, at the same time trying to avoid the flailing hind legs. Down she went, and landed with what is a unique noise – *a bovine thud*. This is the resonant echo from inside the cavernous spaces of the rumen and lungs subsequent to leather, muscle and sturdy bone hitting something solid. Duncan peered over the edge. The cow got up, teetered a little and sauntered away. She did not even bother to look back.

Into the fifties of the number tested, and still the cows were jumping on gates and succeeding in bending down all the top bars of them. By now at least nine cows had escaped from our well-planned system, and we had retrieved them from various parts of the building. At this stage some vets are tempted to begin to count the number of cows left to test. I knew this to be a fatal manoeuvre. The test is not complete until the last one is bled. Until that moment everything is speculation. All went quiet and no cows came forward. I went up to the byre to see what was happening. In one corner of the byre, there was Iain and the two helpers trying to move along an Aberdeen Angus cow. She did not attack them but had something else on her mind. She was upset, judging by her flared nostrils and the way her eyes were not blinking but opening and closing with a violent clicking noise. She had spotted a window about ten feet up the wall. This was her route of escape. So she continually tried to jump up the wall and out of the window… It was an extraordinary sight. We stood back and watched as the cow tried to scramble up the wall.

'Hang on!' I said. 'They usually do not like the smell of a vet. I'll come down there and maybe she will move away.' I went down, skirted round her and moved along the wall. She stopped, saw me, took a deep breath, snorted and moved away up to the exit. There was relief all round. She almost danced into the crush. We quickly sampled her and moved her out as fast as possible.

The next cow came in and then started to reverse backward,

slowly shuffling her feet. Iain stood right behind her, and placing his hand on the gates beside him, tried to push her forward. She slowly pushed him back, so he released his grip and tried again, holding on to another set of gates.

This stopped her a little, but then she applied more force and began to push Iain back again. He rested his grip this time on a breeze block which was part of the masonry of the building. My eyes opened wide as I saw the cow pushing Iain. He was not moving, but the breeze block was. The mortar began to crumble and the brick began to loosen. Other bricks above began to rock a little. Iain relaxed his grip, took a pace or two back, and let the cow turn and retreat. He would get her later.

We were in the sixties now, and while it was obvious that we were near the end, each cow needed individual attention, with about three people guiding, coaxing and prodding it into the crush.

'That's it!' said Duncan.

I looked up and saw Iain and the others walking down towards us. This time they were standing straight-backed and walking with large straight paces. All morning they had been moving round swiftly with their heads down, almost hunched into their shoulders, their legs spaced well apart and their arms ready for balance in case any cow suddenly barged them and put them down on the ground. Cows also tend to react better if your eyes and face are almost on their level; so often you find yourself half bent, trying to guide them away.

We all looked at each other and smiled ruefully. I wiped my hands clean.

'Well, that's done and no one was hurt. All the beasts in one piece. Thank you for your help. It was a bit tricky today. In fact, I haven't done a test like that for a while.' I volunteered this as if to fill the silence. They sucked in at their teeth in half agreement and nodded. They escorted me to the car as I carried my precious cargo of blood tubes. The sixty-five tubes I had collected would hardly fill half a shoebox. When I looked at those tubes with their dark red contents I often wondered if anyone at the receiving laboratory had any idea of the effort and risks taken to obtain the samples.

'Here are the most recent movement records.' Duncan gave

me three pieces of crumpled A4. 'They are printouts from my computer. The Ministry accepts them.'

'Oh, fine. Thanks,' I said, and examined them briefly. Many farmers now used home computers to keep all their records. On occasion the computer looked out of place in an old farm building, but its practical use was its *raison d'être*.

'It is a bit late. Do you want to stop for some soup?' asked Duncan. This placed me in a predicament. Normally I would say yes, and it was a welcome invitation. But today I needed to get away fast.

'Sorry, I had better dash. I am hoping to leave early this afternoon and drive down to relations,' I replied lamely.

'Okay, fine,' Duncan assured me. 'See you, perhaps next time they will be quieter.' And he beamed at me.

Driving away, I saw them exchanging brief comments as in one body they headed for the farmhouse door. They were a dependable group. When events had begun to get difficult they had merely resolved to be silent and tough and continue until the job was done with no panic. It was definitely a Scottish characteristic.

Neil came into the surgery back from his lunch as I began to pack the blood tubes into their protective box prior to posting. He wiped the remains of something delicious from his mouth and said, 'Just back? Problems?' All vets are little jealous of their competence and I had learnt a stock reply from him.

'Oh, nothing that Duncan and I couldn't handle.'

He saw me wink. 'Umm, yes… anything in particular?'

'Well, they were a little on edge and jumpy. In fact, I haven't seen cows prance around like that for a while.'

'Ah well, it is done anyway, and you're back in one piece. When you have finished that I would go if I were you. We'll see you Monday. Have a good weekend and take your time – no speeding down that road, ye hear?'

'Sure, fine, thanks.' Soon I had all the tubes packed. All that needed doing was the paperwork, and that was profuse. I said my goodbyes and headed home for a shower and to gather a weekend bag.

At home Maya, the dog, looked at me expectantly. I apologised to her and explained that today I wouldn't be taking her for a run. Now, she never came with me on my rounds. It appeared to me to be poor biosecurity, and besides I was also a little jittery with her presence beside me. On one occasion the family did not tell me that they had just fed her with the remains of an Indian takeaway. At my first call while I was out of the car attending to a calf, Maya emptied her stomach and bowels over the passenger seat, the floor and under her seat. I had to return to the practice; the car windows all wound down. The mess inside the car had been indescribable. Emma had come out and insisted in helping me tidy it up. Vomitus and excrement had instilled itself into crannies of the car I had not known of. It is possible that that single assistance by Emma convinced me that she is one of the few people in the world with a diamond character.

'Sorry, Maya g-t-g!' Internet shorthand had come into our house. 'Perhaps the others will take you for a run.'

Maya wagged her tail. Her ears hung down and she looked at the end of her nose, a picture of canine melancholy. I trotted to the car and away.

Chapter Four

Long Day's Journey Into Night.

Eugene O'Neill, 1888–1953

The beauty of the Renault Laguna is its deceptive pace. The car is very comfortable and smooth to run. The first time I took Neil for a spin I found him gripping the armrest tight and lifting his knee in anticipation of a crash. That was his hint for me to check the speedometer.

I had left Inverden's wooded glens and in no time I was south of Edinburgh and heading for England down the fast main roads of the Scottish Borders. It was dark and the rain had stopped, the clouds cleared. In these lighting conditions everything appeared sharp and well defined. At the side of the road the precise, continuous, white-paint bands which curved round every corner defined the edges. Most people would find this view from behind the wheel of a car dull, but to me it always had the freshness someone would feel if he had just left prison. (I had been to boarding schools, so this was a concept I was familiar with.) The precise accurate paint marks on the road, the hatched lines zipping past in a rhythmic fashion, the green or red catseyes coming and going, always fascinated me.

My first recollections of roads at night were in the tropics. There, the roads had hidden dangers. There were no markings to guide you, just a black or brown track with potholes which came up on you with no warning. There were few clues as to where the edge of the road lay. Only on hill roads small piles of stones marked the true edge. Occasionally the vehicle would lurch as a wheel found the shifting gravel at the edge of the road. Insects by the thousand and bats by the hundred would rise up and form sparkling showers of gold in the headlights. A mortuary of insects would build up on the windscreen. Only a large jolt caused by a pothole would clear it. You couldn't see the stars by looking out to the front, and if you looked behind the dust often hid them from view. Now and then a magnificent green reflection from the retina of an animal would cause the driver to slow down, and by the time anyone had refocused the mammal had gone. The ride was usually rough and tiring. In contrast, the smooth accuracy of these Scottish mainroads delighted me after the purgatory of my early days.

A series of long straights came up. The car shot down them. As the mid-road markings flowed under the car, I increased speed and was reminded off another part of my childhood – the constant flying. My father had worked abroad and we had travelled after him to all parts of the globe in many different planes, ranging from Dakota DC3s to 747 jumbos. We had taken off from many airstrips in hot countries, and the visual similarities with this main road intrigued me. In the middle distance, representing the developed world, was the tarmac, with all its special markings and lights relevant to fast modern transport. Immediately outside the tarmac was an area of ground lit by my headlights, which would in an aeroplane have been lit by the wing light. Here, where the modern world ended, tussocks of yellow and green grass could be seen representing the undeveloped world. These tussocks would be blowing about in the breeze as if waving goodbye. Lights from small dwellings passed by my car. At the airstrips of my childhood, further away from the tarmac we often saw naked light bulbs lighting up little shanty houses.

There lived those who had not received the benefit of development. These lights produced scenes bursting with deep shadows and highlights which made the mundane articles of life in the tropics beautiful: bicycles; pots; pans; half-dressed children; men in underpants, faces lit only on one side; dilapidated ovens; bottles of beer; religious paintings and ornaments; clothes; electric fans and radios were all on view, but bewitched by these light bulbs swaying in the tropical breeze. My brothers and I would be pressing our noses against the window glass straining to get a better view. At the same time we tried to stop our breath causing condensation which would spoil the picture of the world on the other side of the perimeter fence. We often wondered what tales they all had to tell of their lives, which were so different from our lucky existence. We did not think of ourselves as privileged, but lucky! We could not express the term space-time continuum, yet we thought of these people as being in the same world as ours. But the world also appeared to function in two manners; the small, immediate world we touched now, and another larger world that encompassed all humanity on a vast patchwork blanket which lasted forever.

Every now and then, just as a blanket folds on itself and different parts touch, so we felt every now and then we met and touched another part of this vast sea of immortal people. Our faces would be jerked suddenly from the window at the start of the take-off. As the plane hurried down the runway we would catch a glimpse of some of the huts we had seen before. A slight sadness entered us, as we knew we would not see those people ever again. They were people like us, and so we thought of them as part of our world. Then the plane would be up. Straining our necks around a corner, we looked back through the narrow rear window. All we could see of the naked light bulbs was a string of small diamond lights studded across a dark oblivion.

A main road changed to a more suburban mode as I entered one of the Border towns. A series of shops selling tourist items appeared well lit in the gloom. I parked by one and went in for a cup of coffee. All the souvenirs and woollen clothes were well laid out and a little tempting. However, I examined one or two of them carefully and assessed what they would make in the auction rooms in Inverden. Almost certainly a trifling amount, and that exposed their real value. The buyers at Inverden auction rooms were a tough lot in a good Aberdonian tradition. The auctioneer once complained when they refused to buy silver above scrap metal price. In this Borders shop part of the value was perhaps the romance of Scotland. My coffee had no romance, being hot and strong. It sufficed and would keep me awake. The shop was almost empty. A few folk wandered morosely over the thickly-carpeted floor space fingering goods, while traditional Scottish ballads sunk into all the wool and left a rather dull note. I felt sorry for the staff with so little to do on a night like this. I quickly left for the car; there was no entertainment in watching the dreary shop.

My company now consisted of a CD of *The Gondoliers* by Gilbert and Sullivan. This was another throwback to my past. Dad had carried a small selection of classical music around with him to play on an old Philips reel-to-reel tape recorder. He had a fairly typical selection, but not so nauseating as some of the popular classical radio favourites. We had no Vivaldi *Four Seasons*, no Hummel trumpet pieces, no *Sorcerer's Apprentice*, no flower duet by Delibes, no Mozart Clarinet Concerto. The *1812* was absent; the Toccata and Fugue in D minor also did not make it into the tea chests for foreign parts. Instead, Dad had packed a middle-of-the-road selection even more predictable than classical radio, but far more digestible: all the Beethoven symphonies, a few Brahms, Schubert, Mendelssohn and Schumann symphonies, a few Beethoven piano sonatas, violin concertos by Beethoven, Mendelssohn, Bruch and Tchaikovsky, piano concertos by Beethoven, Brahms, Chopin and Mozart; the Bach *Brandenburg Concerti*; and Handel's *Fireworks*, *Water Music*, concerti grossi and organ concertos. He also had Elgar's *Enigma Variations*, accompanied by a lot of Gilbert and Sullivan. Those were the ones I could remember from days in the tropics

When you had listened to one piece of Dad's music you had had a meal. Present day Classic FM appeared to be a constant stream of hors d'oeuvres; small musical pills to treat mild depression, boredom or stress. Then all those years ago in the tropics we had had the time to hear a whole piece. Late in the evening, Dad's music would float out from the house across the veranda and over the grass towards the plantation's dark cocoa trees. Into those black spaces the music disappeared. In that darkness the sounds of these classics would be drowned by the music of crickets and frogs. I had learnt this when I had had the courage to walk into the cocoa trees. There in the shadows I was surrounded by the loud mystic noises of countless invisible insects, frogs, toads, and small running mammals near me. As I emerged from the shades of the foliage the bright lights of the house would appear, accompanied by softer reflections coming from the grass. Then, just as my feet touched the grass at the edge of the trees, the music of Schubert or some other great would reach me faintly. It was a surreal experience. One turn back to the trees and all my ears could pick up was the sounds of dark, raw nature. Turn again back to the house, and the bright lights with the enticing music from the frail tape recorder beckoned me home.

The music from the Gilbert and Sullivan CD teased my thoughts. A phrase came by: 'But stay – the present and the future – they are another's; but the past that at least is ours, and none can take it from us. As we may revel in naught else, let us revel in that!'

It was always tempting to dream of the past. I considered that WS Gilbert had been no fool, but the present for me had immediate demands. Suddenly I found myself cornering violently as the road twisted down the rain-soaked hills into some small valleys. Norbury lay in one of them. Some '30 MPH' signs came up. A pub passed by, followed by a couple of houses, and then darkness. Three miles later and I caught sight of a simple white sign. A small red crest topped it and underneath the title 'NORBURY'. There was no outward sign that Norbury was twinned with some other European town or that it was in 'THE VALE OF NORTHUMBRIA', or that it was a five-star sight for tourism. For all I knew, it had these titles but in an old English way it understated its importance. Two hundred yards further on and the street lights appeared, revealing not a pavement but a wide grass verge with intermittent driveways which led into gaps in the high beech hedge. The verges broke down to pavement on either side. No one was out; the weather was foul. Barriers appeared between the road and the pavement. This was a hint of the presence of schoolchildren: even they weren't out and about tonight. Consistent with the intimation of a school, several large gothic buildings reared up on either side. I felt as though I was driving down a parting sea with wave crests in castellated outlines looking down on me. No light emanated from the high vertical walls of the school. Then the shape of the buildings changed and lights came out of small porthole windows. The shape of the roofs changed into complex twisted filigree shapes. I stopped my car at a set of red pedestrian lights. A car wedged between two Dreadnoughts in dry dock would have had a similar view.

This was Norbury College. The school inside these ironclad

walls had been regimented. A complement of over a thousand people was mustered and checked daily. Bells rang, quiet periods were regulated, drills performed, discipline maintained and punishments meted out. Yet, with the exception of one subject, I had enjoyed this college. A determined streak in me had revelled in taking the rough with the smooth. The comradeship of beating the system had always kept me alive, minute by minute, in a reality lacking in the outside world. In my rational moments I would never want to go back and start again at Norbury College – the school where I had to queue daily for rations of bread and milk, lock away in secret places my best possessions, and hope that the most recent cold bath was my last. But… with the same comrades and company, I would be tempted to chance my arm again.

Suddenly I had left the school behind. On my left, surrounded by old gravestones spaced across a well-kept lawn, stood a typical perpendicular-style English country church. Spotlights from the lawn highlighted the Irish green of the grass, the yellow dots of drizzle descending, the texture of the sandstone church walls and a limp flag of St George that was twisted round about a short flagpole at the top of the tower. This was an England I expected. The road curved round two sides of the church ground and then opened out into the wide main street of Norbury. Here the market street was undiminished by the weather. The black road sparkled from the light given out by a series of baroque-style street lamps which lined up in the centre and either side of the street. A few people in genderless overcoats were walking quickly along the sides. Their shoulders were hunched and they skipped to dodge the puddles. The majority were sensibly snug in a pub, the signs of which were dotted down the street and on occasion caught the lights as they swung wildly in the wind.

I drove to the left of the town hall. It stood at the end of this market street. Its solid pillars overshadowed a wide arcade that encircled it. At the college we had often lounged against these pillars, chatting across arches to all and sundry. Although I could not see it I knew there to be an ornate crest on one side and a clock with hourly moving burgher men on the other. It was a style of civic design that would appeal to a more Germanic nature than mine.

My destination was to be found up a small lane beyond the town hall. My car nosed up a side lane. Creepers hung down from high red-brick walls, which narrowed the lane a little. I drove past with care. The creepers moved in the wind, showering the ground below with their own special tears. The walls disappeared to be replaced by low white fences protecting petite gardens. Aunt Sarah's garden was silhouetted by the lights from her house. She had switched on every light bulb in the house. Perhaps she was concerned that my memory might have faded. How she could have thought that? As a schoolboy I had yearned to go there for food and company. I parked the car as close as I could to the fence. A gust of wet air rushed into the car as I got out. As quickly as possible, I ran to the front door with my case. There was no time to admire her thatched cottage with its white walls and lead-laced glass windows. I tapped on the door and noticed something resembling a large pillow move off the window sill.

'Oh, Richard, Richard dear, come in, come in!' A delighted Aunt Sarah hauled me inside. She slammed the door shut to stop more autumn leaves following me in. 'There now, we are all in for the night. How are you?'

'I'm fine, Aunt Sarah.' We were always formal at first in our family. 'How about you?'

'Well… what do you think?' and she stood a few paces away from me.

'Oh, I think she has the fine body of a woman.' I quoted in a bombastic tone.

Aunt Sarah recognised my line from Gilbert and Sullivan. 'Oh, you beast!' she replied, hitting the air in mock frustration. 'Now I don't know what to think.'

'Stop!' I directed. 'Take another pace back, please.' I took a long look.

'Ah,' she murmured. 'The vet at work—'

I did not let her complete her sentence. 'Silence… this takes me a couple of seconds more.' I stared. She was well preserved, I had to admit. She had kept her black hair long, though now it was flecked with grey. Her face was oval-shaped with high cheekbones – the high cheekbones beloved of all Chinese and found in the women of Shanghai. There were no wrinkles on her face and her eyes were clear and dark brown. Only a minute amount of make-up had been applied. She was neither fat nor thin, but a thick tweed skirt probably hid a long fit figure.

'You are still beautiful,' I observed. 'But please don't ask me again or you will embarrass both of us.'

'Fine, I can trust my nephew.' She relaxed visibly. 'Come in and say hello to Wooihfung and Nganhong.' These were her embarrassing names for her cats – the Cantonese for the Hong Kong and Shanghai Bank. My uncle had met Sarah in China when they both worked as juniors in the bank. They had married out there. Mixed marriages weren't too uncommon. They had come back to Britain, where my uncle had started as a teacher at Norbury College. He had died unexpectedly a few months after Sarah had given birth to twin baby girls. It was a difficult time for her. Luckily the school generously gave her my uncle's tied house to live in and advised her on how to bring up the twins. They also assisted her in securing a job as a part-time librarian. In typical Chinese fashion, she threw herself into this role and now she was as British in behaviour as anyone. This was not a tacky imitation on her part but a true assimilation of all our mores. She had the talent of a chameleon. The only difference was the Chinese grace she brought to many English customs.

She called the cats, and so they appeared; two enormous long-haired felines. They were crosses because they did not have the short noses of Persians. Both were overweight in a grandiose fashion. Wooihfung must have been the 'pillow' I had seen falling off the window sill. He was an enormous football of fur walking toward me with a mincing gait.

'Goodness, how much does he weigh?' I asked. 'He must be at least six kilos.'

'He is seven and a half,' observed my aunt. 'It is one of my few indulgences. Fat cats and slim owner.' Aunt Sarah stood at ease as Wooihfung sidled up to and started stroking his side against her leg. His eyes were bright yellow and suggested a wicked streak in him in spite of his soft exterior.

'Anyway, you might need a bite,' she declared. 'Put your case down here at the foot of the stairs and follow me. I have a little surprise for you.'

I followed her into the kitchen, bending my head to dodge some of the low beams. The table was laid in red and chopsticks were evident. In the middle was a bottle of Rémy Martin.

'Oh, this could be good,' I acknowledged. I changed my speech to some basic Cantonese. 'Some Chinese food. You are spoiling me!'

'Oh yes,' said Aunt Sarah in Cantonese. Hers was a little rusty too since she naturally spoke Shanghaienese or Mandarin. The Hong Kong dialect was truly her fourth language, after English. 'I thought after your time in Hong Kong you might like some dim sum. I apologise it is the wrong time of day. But these Amoy ones are very good for food bought in Europe.'

She produced from her oven some wicker dim sum baskets and opened them out across the table. There were the usual suspects – *chasiubau, hagauu, fangwo, ngauyuhk* and some other exotics.

'*Msai haakhai!*' she shouted. 'No formality!' And on her cue I took up my chopsticks and dived in. I was interested to see if she had managed to produce something close to the food I had enjoyed in Hong Kong. She saw me slowly chewing the pork bun. Yes, it was good.

'*Ho sik.* Very good,' I murmured in Cantonese. Pleased, she grabbed the bottle of brandy and poured a generous helping into my glass. For a few minutes we revelled in recreating the happy family atmosphere of a Chinese meal, occasionally grabbing a titbit and placing it on another's plate. Then I saw Aunt Sarah pause a little with a shrimp dumpling in her sticks.

'Something the matter?' I asked.

'Yes and no,' she replied in English. I straightened up from my rice bowl. 'It is not possible to explain in Chinese. This brings back a memory. Perhaps you will be appalled or laugh at me. You are after all a vet.' I braced myself for some terrible confession. She carried on.

'About three weeks ago I was in the garden pruning all the roses and preparing the garden for winter when Wooihfung ran past me into the house. Nothing too extraordinary in that – even he occasionally tries to be athletic. But then Mrs Simmonds came rushing down at me, very, very angry. She was screaming and crying. Her daughter came and joined her too, very upset. They told me that they were used to Wooihfung coming to visit and they sometime gave him a little food, but usually made him go politely. However they had found him in the kitchen. He had opened their gerbil cage and was helping himself to the little baby gerbils that had been born a few days before. When they shouted at Wooihfung he had rushed past them with one little gerbil between his jaws! They tried to tackle him and had missed. Now they were down to catch him. So I immediately ran into the house and grabbed the murderer, but there was nothing Mrs Simmonds and I could see.'

'Aunt Sarah,' I commented gently, 'I don't see the connection between this and the *hagauu*...'

'Yes, well, you see,' explained Aunt Sarah, 'we decided to see if Wooihfung had dropped the little gerbil while making his escape. But then I did not know what we were looking for. So Mrs Simmonds and her daughter took me to the cage and showed me the two remaining newborn gerbils. They were grey and shiny with a suggestion of pink inside.' I looked at the *hagaau*. The light grey skin of the dumpling surrounded the hint of pink of the shrimp inside. Now I could see the resemblance.

'Oh, I see. That does put a slightly different edge on it,' I added sympathetically. 'Still, Wooihfung is a natural killer. Most cats are. You did attempt to stop that by the grossly excessive amount of food you give him. Did you find the baby gerbil?'

'No, and I did not know what to do in compensation.' She looked genuinely concerned. 'In the end I went and had a chat with Mr Simmonds. He looked very serious at first. He is a forest ranger. Then he looked round slyly, just like this...' Here Aunt Sarah slid her eyes back and forth like a wicked Dame in a Christmas Pantomime. 'And he then just burst out laughing. So I was very confused. He said he didn't really like rodents; they ruined most of his work. He suggested I give his daughter a box of chocolates. Oh, it is very difficult to know how people will behave in England when it comes to animals.'

'Now, that is a true comment, Aunt Sarah,' I said, to encourage her. 'You entered a veritable minefield and have come away unscathed. Here, more brandy to steady your nerves before you have your next *hagau* – and it is *not* a little gerbil.' Aunt Sarah looked relieved that the animal professional had not condemned her. Gingerly she nibbled at her dim sum.

'Another?' She offered me some more brandy. Seeing me hesitate, she continued. 'There are no rules for you to break now.'

I raised my eyebrows in assent. She filled my glass. Aunt Sarah was referring to the first few of her infamous meals given when I was at school at Norbury College. She had invited me to bring some friends out from school for Sunday lunch. A friend was looking after her twins for the day. On the first occasion we had all eaten far too much after only three courses. We were surprised when she had said there were five more courses to come. As innocents, we had confessed that we had already had a lot. 'No problem,' she said, 'take a short walk up the hill and back, take your time, you will find the food will settle and you can manage the rest.' We had taken her advice, and sure enough, pacing ourselves we had completed the standard eight-course Chinese meal. However, on return to school three of my five friends had been gloriously sick. The school Sister had been worried that a bug had just arrived at school. Investigations were carried out and the common denominator of my Aunt's excessive generosity was identified. Nothing was said.

At the second meal Aunt Sarah converted to British fare. Only four courses were offered this time: Scotch broth, roast beef, Yorkshire pudding and the gastronomic accessories, rhubarb crumble and ice cream, finished off with cheeses and fruit. The latter was a particular sacrifice, since like so many of her countrymen she did not like cheese. As a sop to the lack of courses (and besides, four was an unlucky Chinese number), she had also added in Irish coffee and gave us beer to drink. She had suddenly realised that she had six inebriated teenagers on her hands. She had panicked and in desperation had locked the door and refused to allow us back to school until we had sobered up. A stream of black coffees was given us and around five p.m., with a slight dose of the shakes but very contented, we rolled back to school. The incident – in particular my aunt's afternoon kidnap of five innocent school children – got out. Poor Aunt Sarah was scared when the Head invited himself to her house.

The Head insisted that she prepare nothing in the way of food and drink for him. He was merciless. Aunt Sarah later recounted two sentences that she recollected with clarity: 'You do realise that the college would have a serious problem if anyone found out that their son had been kidnapped, albeit temporarily, by a Chinese lady short of funds? Some of the more sensitive parents might think that a member of the Triads had come to work at Norbury.'

Aunt Sarah was genuinely worried that they would take back her tied house. The Head was fair but firm. He reassured her that the house was safe as it was given on the strength of her husband's tragic death. However, he had a few guidelines to suggest which he asked her to abide by. Two days later I was summoned to the Headmaster's office. This was the only time I went there. He usually communed with heads of houses, prefects, masters and so on. He explained the 'ground rules' to Aunt Sarah's luncheon parties: no more than five courses; no more than one pint of beer or equivalent; guests to be back by four thirty and to obtain prior permission from the housemaster. Only two such 'gaudies', as he referred to them, were to be allowed per term. I was asked if I had any comments. I replied, 'No, sir... thank you, sir.' These were the only words I ever spoke to the Headmaster.

Later I came close to him at prize giving, but then only received a beaming smile. The words on that occasion came from the dignitary handing out the prize for biology – that being the only subject I displayed any genuine talent in.

'Those were the days,' I murmured, looking at my glass and the brandy turning inside it. 'Those meals were incredible. In fact I had a problem because folk kept on asking me if they could come. I could have made myself very popular with one or two important boys if I'd let them visit.'

'But you didn't,' she said, smiling. 'I noticed that. You always used to tell me if a different friend was coming and explain why one of the original five was not up to it. You were very particular about that; it was touching. Perhaps you did not know I have had one or two come here since then.' She winked.

'Who, Aunt Sarah? You never!' I sounded shocked.

She tapped her nose. 'No names, no pack drill. They came with girlfriends for me to check. Well, to vet really. Part of the deal was that I would never tell. So there.' She looked straight ahead.

'No, come on! Who was it – Alex, Tudor or James?'

'Don't even ask,' she rounded on me. 'Besides, I think you brought your Jill here for a weekend.'

'Ah, that was just to meet the family,' I said lamely. 'Okay, yes, I remember I did ask you what you thought. Did all the others do the same?'

'There you are, at it again! I won't tell you how many came. Yes, but those who did come wanted my opinion. I even went to one of the weddings, and the girl said she had been terrified of being the recipient of "the curse of Sarah"!'

'No, really?' I was desperately trying to work out who it could be.

'Anyway, she need not have worried,' said Aunt Sarah meaningfully.

I decided to change the subject. 'How are the twins?'

'Fine, fine. They phone now and then. The birds have flown now. You know they both work in London after graduating? Merchant bankers, both of them: very Chinese, I suppose. They are not money-grabbing, you know, but they like to have it around.' She paused and I could see the implied self-criticism. Money had been tight when she had brought them up. 'I think your mother sees more of them than I do. She is just a short train journey away and they enjoy spoiling your father.'

Once again I could see the worry – the concern that they had hardly known their own father, and so mine was a type of substitute they could visit and enjoy. Besides, my dad could really act the grumpy, humorous and lovable man. 'Well, I am here,' I murmured.

'Of course you are, Richard. I am jealous not of other members of the family. It is geography I hate. I suppose I wish they were a little closer. They do come and see me. Jemimah was here only two weeks ago. My Gohd!' (She had resorted to the Chinese pronunciation of God putting an 'h' in with the 'o'.) 'I am going to become a jealous old witch if I don't look out.' Her eyes flashed at me. Suddenly I could see the potential too.

'Well, we do not want that. If there is anything I can do to help, just tell me, won't you?' I replied blithely.

Without a break she said, 'I will. I can hold you to that.'

'Yes...' I hesitated for a fraction, considered what the worst was that my aunt could get up to, and repeated, 'Yes, if there is anything I can do to help, I will.'

She looked happy.

'Good. I am glad.' I wondered what was happening. She sat up a little. 'Yes, that is what family is for, isn't it? Anyway, we must plan tomorrow. You usually like a rake through the Norbury bookshops and stalls, don't you? Yes, well, by the weekend books I have seen enough of, so I will let you have two hours of that, as per our usual agreement; and then we head for Newcastle. I don't have tickets for the game.'

'Oh.' I was surprised; she was a diehard Newcastle United fan. I knew one of her recent prize possessions to be a shirt signed by Alan Shearer. She would never allow anyone in the family to ask how much it cost.

'Instead, a friend has arranged for us to go to a hospitality suite for BP executives.' She smirked.

'Magic!' I beamed.

'I thought you would be pleased. It is okay – I do know one or two of them. I keep back books for them when they are desperate and so on.'

My eyes began to close a little. Seeing this, she took charge. 'You, young boy, must go to bed. We will get you up there now, your usual room.'

I protested without conviction. The brandy had mellowed me. My aunt and I slowly went up the steps, she carrying Nahnhong, and his tail swished out from below the crook of her elbow. I followed, pulling up my case. At the end of the corridor was my usual room with the bathroom door opposite. She opened the door and I went in.

'Goodnight, I will wake you at a civilised hour.' Aunt Sarah so loved phrases from other spheres.

I saw her disappear down the corridor, her long hair flowing a little off her shoulders. I nipped into the bathroom, had a quick shower and collapsed into the bed, which was set against a bow window. The bed was ancient with a dip in the middle and bolster pillows. Two or three people could hide inside it. It was like a warm cave. Soon I was asleep.

Chapter Five

That's the classical mind at work, runs fine inside but
looks dingy on the surface.

RT Pirsig, *Zen and the Art of Motorcycle Maintenance*

A cat purred in my ear. I lay motionless and gathered my
thoughts. Slowly I rotated my head and peered over the
bedclothes. Something was so close to me that I couldn't focus on
it. It was white. One of the two, I thought, pulling my head back
and realigning my eyes. Opposite each of my squinting eyes
Woouihfung's own half-opened eyes surveyed me.

'Oh, hello, Wooih,' I greeted him. 'Good morning, *Jo san.*' I
said in Cantonese and offered to stroke him. He raised himself,
stretched and retreated to the far corner of the bed. Then I
noticed that Nganhong was in the opposite far corner. They
watched me like two celestial guardians stationed at the end of my
bed. A tap on the door preceded my Aunt's head.

'Ah, I see they have woken you up. I let them into your room
a while ago. They kept on scratching at the door. Perhaps it was
your snoring that interested them. Anyway, here is some tea.
Breakfast in half an hour.' She advanced across the room with the
tray. Her half-dried hair was laid across the front of one shoulder
on top of her long silk gown. The cats, in response to her
entrance, jumped down and left. I placed the tray with teapot,
cup, milk jug, sugar cubes and tongs on the window ledge. It
fitted neatly on to the ledge, which was contiguous with the edge
of my bed.

'Sleep well?'

'Yes, fine. Not even a headache.'

'That is good brandy for you,' she laughed and left.

This twenty-minute period before getting up was one of the
great luxuries of life. Morning tea, a bow window and a garden to

enjoy from a warm bed amounted to a luxury I doubted princes enjoyed often.

Thirty minutes later I was washed and shaved and down in the kitchen. We had a sparse breakfast of toast and marmalade. Aunt Sarah appeared preoccupied in the papers and intent on sending me out on the book trail.

'If you go to Halkett's bookshop, ask for Luke. I have asked him to hold on to one or two things for you. Take some money. Be back by eleven forty-five, as we must leave then. James is joining us.'

'James?' I was surprised.

'Yes, he is a chemistry teacher at the college. The person who often comes along with me is busy, and so he has stepped in. I like him and hope you will too. Anyway, no point in wasting a good ticket,' she explained. My Aunt often had odd plans so I left it unquestioned.

Market days had always been Wednesdays and Saturdays in Norbury. The stalls set themselves up in the middle of the wide main street in place of a central car park. By the light of day I now had a good sight of the town hall at one end of the street. The large perpendicular-style church at the other end acted as a cover for Norbury College. I browsed my way though a bookstall and occasionally listened in on the passing comments of town folk and public school boys. Then I came face to face with a man whose visage was indelibly impressed on my mind. He looked straight at me. I was riveted to the ground unable to run away. Transfixed, I tried a diplomatic escape.

'Hello, sir,' I said. The old man looked harder at me while holding on to a book balanced on a pile of paperbacks.

'I doubt you remember me, Dr Leasden. You taught me Classics at the college.' I nodded in the direction of the church.

'That stands to reason, since I only taught Classics and I was at the college for thirty years. Rather, tell me your name and house.'

'Jones, Richard Jones, Shaftesbury House.' The old man froze.

'Yes, I do recollect you. After all, my, you have changed. You hold a unique place in my teaching career. The only pupil I insisted drop Greek. Is that not correct, Jones?' His thick grey eyebrows went up and down twice as though he was scoring points in some sport.

'I think I can remember your final oration to me.' I took a deep breath and quoted: 'Yes, you, Jones, have impressed me with the length of time it has taken you to learn the Greek alphabet. While it is common to say that someone lacks talent, this is not so in your case. To state that you have a disability to study Greek would be an insult to the capacities of the lame, the halt and the blind. You have an ability to terrorise the Greek language. Your completed Greek prose is so destructive that I am forced, for light relief, to meditate upon the freshly smouldering lava-smothered ruins of Pompeii. Your Greek unseen, Jones, is so unseen that it is easier to detect the lost city of Atlantis. The Head and I have agreed that you cease forthwith to study the subject. I will ensure, so long as God gives me breath, that you pass Latin "O" level. Greek will always be Greek to you, Jones. You may leave the classroom now.'

I paused and added, 'You see, I remember. Even today I still remember the shocked silence as I left the scholars classroom with my head down.'

'Perhaps I was a little severe on you. You cannot get away with that now.' Briefly he too looked down at his feet.

How right he was! That single incident was the talk of the school for a week and spawned a cottage industry of new nicknames for me: 'El Greco', 'Up Pompeii', 'The Omega Factor', 'Disability Jones' and 'Classical Dick' were some that I could recollect.

'But I credit myself,' he continued, looking up, 'in steering you away from the rocks of the Classics and into the calm waters of the sciences. You did well at sciences, did you not?'

'Yes, you were correct, sir. I am now a vet. Went up to Oxbridge and so on.'

'And so on,' he mimicked me in a benign way. We were obviously past enmity now. 'A vet, hmmm... I wonder if I could ask you a few questions?' He saw my worried look.

'No, no, not about a particular case. I am more interested in principles, reason and logic. Why don't we go to the Copper Kettle and have a cup of tea? My shout.'

'Veterinary principles?'

'Yes, Jones, strictly veterinary.'

'Fine. Why not?' Here at last was my one opportunity to run a ring or two round this old teacher. At least I could restore a counter-argument to his view that I was an exotic boffin or some sort of academic terrorist. We crossed out of the centre of the street into the tearooms.

'Now, Jones, I want to ask you about TSEs. I have been reading the subject up and it has interested me.' He saw my surprise.

'Even classicists can use the Internet to study. But you give me the opportunity for some first-hand input.' He drew me towards a suitable table.

'You mean the diseases – scrapie, BSE, CJD, new variant CJD?' I asked, in an attempt to find out at what level this discussion was going to take place.

'Yes, yes – all those and kuru, CWD et cetera.' He looked excited.

'Well, fire away,' I said. 'I am not an expert but I have a feel for the subject.'

The waitress arrived.

'Cream tea for two, please. I am retired and Richard here is, as far as I can see, not on duty. Ergo, we need spoiling.' I wondered if he had used Latin out of consideration for my Greek catastrophies.

'Well, let me see. The appearance of BSE was a new phenomenon was it not?' he queried.

'Oh yes. Quite a surprise.'

'So with this new situation – a new disease in cattle – were you expecting any other new surprises?' he asked innocuously.

'What do you mean?' I fished a bit. 'I think there was some basic surveillance added.'

'Well, if it is was a new disease, different, it should not have been too great a surprise if on occasion it went to man or some other species? After all, that seems to have been unexpected. I recollect senior civil servants on many occasions telling us there was no problem.'

'Yes, that was a surprise. A nasty shock, in fact. You see, because scrapie is a similar disease and doesn't appear to cause disease in man we did not expect BSE to go to man,' I explained.

'But BSE is not scrapie,' he countered. 'There is no evidence that it is scrapie, is there?'

'None at all,' I agreed. 'Some people say it is a mutant scrapie, but it is definitely different from all previously known strains of scrapie.'

'So to use scrapie as a model for BSE was, on reflection, incorrect?' he added.

'Well, yes, as an exact model. But we had nothing else to go on.'

'But you had all the other TSEs to use as possible models.'

'I agree,' I said, looking in my teacup and concentrating hard. 'But as far as I know none of them is BSE. In fact we still do not know where BSE came from. There are prions of one form or other all over the place.'

There was a pause.

'So now, with scrapie, I gather the government is intent to eradicate it.' His eyebrows rose a fraction in interrogation.

'Yes.'

'Scrapie is a disease that we have known about for hundreds of years – and does no harm to man?' The eyebrows had raised a fraction higher. Too late I began to recollect his admiration for the Socratic method.

'Yes.'

'When you eradicate it, if you succeed, then a new situation will occur, will it not?'

'I am not sure what you are driving at,' I said.

'Well, correct me if I am wrong, Richard, but for hundreds of years you, I and all our ancestors have been exposed to scrapie. After all, veganism is relatively rare and recent in our culture. Now you are proposing that we should no longer be exposed to a benign prion.'

'Yes, well, it does no wrong. We don't know what it does,' I added calmly.

'You don't know what it does, but you will remove it?' His eyes twinkled as he masticated a cream bun, then he cleared his throat. 'I am so glad you are not the mechanic for my motor car. Has it occurred to you it might do some good?'

'Ah, well it is unlikely that it does any good,' I said hastily.

'Why? Give me a reason?'

'I've none.'

Impasse.

'Have any experiments been performed on pre-exposure to scrapie or other prion agents? This might be a reasonable thing to do.'

'It's funny you say that,' I hurried on, proud that I could remember some experiments. 'Scientists once injected mice with different strains of scrapie. They had different incubation periods. They found if you injected a mouse with – and this is an approximation – an 180-day incubation strain first, followed by a 250-day incubation strain, then the mice went down with the disease after 180 days. But if they injected the 250-day strain first followed by the 180-day strain, the mice went down after 250 days. The first prion in set the incubation period for the appearance of TSE symptoms. I suppose if the first prion in had an incubation period longer than the mouse's life it might not get a TSE but die of old age. Funny, isn't that?' I looked at him.

'Well, it is interesting, but also shows how little we do know.' He leant back. 'So with the advent of BSE we encountered a new relationship between prions and man. That has caused a few problems, wouldn't you say?' I nodded. 'Now, ten years or so later, you are going to eradicate scrapie, and that too will deliberately create a new relationship between prions and man. Yet in both cases you do not know the final outcome...'

'Well, it is something like that. Perhaps you are too concerned. That is my professional opinion,' I said, trying to placate him.

'Agreed, and mine is merely rational deduction.' He smiled. 'Anyway, why the urgency for scrapie eradication?'

'We are unable on clinical grounds to say whether a sheep has scrapie or BSE,' I explained, feeling on safer ground.

'So you decide to do both at once – look for BSE in sheep with more testing and eradicate TSEs at the same time?'

'Oh, yes,' I concurred, not seeing the trap.

'Richard, let me give you an illustration.' He leant forward as though mentioning something indecent. 'I hate illustrations as they always have some weaknesses, but this may help. Suppose you and I are sent as enforcement officers to a large supermarket.

We have been told that there is an unproven possibility of a toxic fungus on the apples. Also that we have definite evidence that there is no toxic fungus on any apples completely coloured yellow or green. In contrast we are told that apples with any red skin might have toxins. I am instructed to eradicate and remove all the at-risk apples. You are instructed to check all the at risk apples for the presence of toxins. What is going to happen?'

'If you start well before me I won't have any apples to test. They're all gone,' I answered tentatively.

'Precisely,' he said. 'And if I manage to have eradicated half the red apples before you arrive, then your survey will have only covered at best fifty per cent of the population. Not a very good survey.'

'Whatever happens,' I ventured, 'the only apples left for the consumers will be the Golden Delicious and the Granny Smiths, a narrow genetic base, and not a great variety. I see your point. We will never know if there was toxin present in the apples; or if we do find it, the full extent of the problem.'

'Do you think there is a lot of BSE in sheep?' He asked. 'Sponge finger?' he proffered a plate to me. I hesitated momentarily but his face gave nothing away.

'Well, here is my opinion with a little reason,' I said, playing again for time. 'All the sheep that could have been infected in the first few years by mouth should be dead by now. Any sheep that have BSE today have either received it from their parents or by whatever means BSE transmits between sheep. This may, and this is opinion, be a low rate of horizontal transmission. Judging by the few cases of scrapie reported or seen, I think the level if present is very low. Culling a lot of sheep will reduce the chances of finding it.'

Leasden nodded in agreement. 'Is the government surveying a lot of sheep?' he asked

'Oh yes, over twenty thousand.'

'What type of sheep is that?'

'Nearly all at the abbatoir.'

'Is scrapie often seen at the abbatoir?' he asked, apparently concentrating on a few crumbs on his plate.

'No, not really, it is a disease of older sheep often in poor condition. "Not much eating on them", as they say. The young healthy sheep rarely have it.'

'So, Richard, ninety-nine per cent of your present search is in the wrong place: not at the older sheep.' The eyebrows now went up and down thrice.

'Well *yes* and *no*. It bolsters consumer confidence. After all it is the young sheep that the consumers eat.'

'But it is the *parents* who might actually have it. It is looking in the wrong place if you want to find the disease, is it not? And how many have definitely been tested to see whether they have scrapie or BSE?'

'Only about two hundred have been definitely checked to differentiate between scrapie and BSE.'

'I am only a classicist, but to me that seems a big difference from your original consumer confidence-boosting figure. *Quis numerus rectum est. Ducenti aut viginti milia?*' He stared at me. I thought for a second.

'Put that way it is not so good. I am not defending them. They are trying their best.'

'Are they? If you want to find out whether a disease is present, when it is at a suspected low level, should you not look in the right place and with massive incentives for reporting? For example, offer one thousand guineas for any sheep that is positive for BSE. Four times market price for a scrapie positive, and two times market price for vet-checked suspects which turn out to be negative.' He opened his hands in a gesture of munificence.

'That is an idea. It might be expensive.'

'As expensive as genetic testing?'

'You have a point, sir,' I said, 'but even after that, what happens with the result of the survey? If we find BSE then there is a problem. The Minister stated he would very likely eradicate the UK flock. That would mean all the previous genetic testing would have been wasted.'

'And if you do not find BSE in spite of massive rewards for finding it, what does that tell you?' He fixed me with his 'tell all' stare.

'There is a very good chance we have not got BSE in sheep.'

'Well *that is* a thought, Jones.' He winked. 'By the way, you thoroughly deserved your Latin "O" level.'

'Yes, I am quite proud of it. It was hard work but worth the effort.'

'I can tell you now that you were one mark above the pass mark, and a pass is a pass. For a scientist it was a good performance.'

'I am impressed with your knowledge of TSEs,' I said, attempting to return the compliment.

'Oh, I just came across it on the Internet and became engrossed. For instance, the government's requirement for the ARR homozygous is fascinating. It appears that by a slow process they want all the sheep to be cloned for three gene loci. Wouldn't sell well at a supermarket – "Cloned for three genes". Sponge cake?' He pushed it toward me. I thought these sponge references might be a little bit in bad taste, and as if divining my thoughts he added, 'Tastes delicious!'

'But these genes give scrapie resistance,' I said. 'Well, that is not quite true,' I corrected myself. 'They give BSE resistance. You can achieve scrapie resistance with other genotypes.'

'Ah, so your genetic policy is for this disease, BSE. You know not what or where it is. How interesting, a disease policy which is in itself a gene-cloning experiment in sheep in order to control a possibly nonexistent disease in sheep.' He was now delicately spreading a scone while he held it well above his plate.

'I say, Mr Leasden, that is little over the top,' I countered.

'I am not so sure, Richard. To be frank, after speaking with you there appears to be more reasoned common sense in Greek mythology than in the practise of state veterinary medicine in Britain. More tea?'

We decided to move on to other less taxing subjects.

'Do you come here often?' Leasden asked. I hesitated; I was not sure I wanted Aunt Sarah involved with him. Then I relented, hoping the truth would save me.

'I am visiting my Aunt. We see each other now and then. Family, and all that,' I said somewhat lamely. I was not going to go into all the details.

'I am sure,' said Leasden, the height of propriety. 'And this afternoon, are you up to anything interesting? I don't imagine you will want to walk through the school grounds. You have already met Banquo's ghost in finding me, and I doubt you will be out for more of the same.'

I was severely tempted to say that he was above the league of Banquo and furthermore I had few other major ghosts to encounter at school.

'You are correct, in fact we are off to watch the Magpies.' I cleaned my plate in schoolboy fashion.

'I see them too, sometimes. Not today, though; other matters. Against Southampton, aren't they? Should be a good match.'

'Yes,' I said plainly. 'In fact I have to get to a shop soon… would you mind me leaving suddenly?'

'Of course, of course. It was kind of you illuminate me on your day off. Have a good day. Perhaps we will meet gain.'

'Yes. I am sure,' I said, shook his hand and left. Out of the corner of my eye I saw Leasden pick up the bill.

I left the tearoom with my head buzzing. On my weekend off to suddenly deal with all those veterinary matters was not settling at all. Damn Leasden. Damn him! I thought. Only he could ruin a day like that. Still, I had been trapped into it. I could simply have said no. But then I thought this had been my one opportunity to put one over him and make him seem small. I thought he would ask me basic questions about canine distemper or cat flu, not the latest data on prions and TSEs. I barged into Halkett's and almost knocked someone over. I apologised off-handedly.

'Steady as you go,' said one of the shop assistants, laughing at me. I bit my tongue again and demanded.

'I am looking for Luke.'

'*Ecce homo*,' he said, stretching out his hands. He saw my withering stare, and immediately commiserated. 'Rough day?'

'No. It was fine until half an hour ago. I met my old Classics teacher.' I amazed myself at my indiscretion, but then I was still fuming.

'Oh, usually I am glad to see them. Just to remind them of the subject I have given up – Classics – and how I am now onto much more interesting things.' Luke walked away. He was about twenty years old, wore glasses and sported slightly long frizzy hair. He reminded me of a postgraduate research student. I followed him down to the dark recesses of the shop. The fact that my Classics master had given up on me rather than me giving up on him was not one I was going to divulge to Luke. He stopped and grabbed some books.

'Your Aunt thought you might like these.' He handed the books to me nonchalantly.

'How did you know it was me?' I said surprised.

'Oh, it's a small town. Everyone knows everyone. You would know that from Scotland.' My eyebrows shot up. 'Number plates,' he continued. 'ASE on a plate is near Aberdeen. I have relatives there. Besides – please accept this as a compliment – you don't smell but there is an aura of a vet about you.' He gazed at me.

'You are brutally frank,' I said.

'But then I know your aunt and have some idea of who she is related to. Your family seems to take things like that on the chin.' This was becoming too close for comfort, so I examined the books.

'Goodness, where did you get these?' I gasped.

'Thought you would like them. I have not had a set like that for ages, and certainly not in such good condition.' Luke scratched the back of his head and admired the set of six books in my hand. They were the *Giles Cartoon Annuals* for the Second World War in almost mint condition. Inside were the comic drawings of Hitler and Mussolini in between those of the Giles family.

'They are genuine and not forgeries. I checked it out myself,' he explained.

'Of course I will take them. How much are you needing for them?' I demanded.

'Fifty pounds.' He saw me hesitate. 'The lot.'

'Yes, yes, fine,' I said, excited. Then I considered what was a ridiculously cheap price. 'Are you sure? It is a bargain at that.'

'Sure, I'm not meant to tell you, but your aunt subsidised the price, as she knew that you, if anyone, should have them. But the other cartoon books,' he pointed at another little pile, 'you're to pay for. You will find the price of all of them inside the flyleaf.'

After a few minutes I had completed my purchases and headed back to Aunt Sarah's. She opened the door as I came in.

'Success?' She cocked her head on one side.

'Yes, yes.' I hurried in. 'I met that beastly Classics master of mine, Leasden… quite upset me. But your books worked magic. They will be great for my collection.' I saw my aunt freeze for a second while looking at the door sill, then she explained.

'Well, I have something else to take you away from any worries. Or perhaps exchange them. Here, grab this.' She handed me a rolled-up towel. 'There are some trunks in there, and we are going off right now to a swimming pool beside St James's Park. This is James. James: Richard, Richard: James. Just wait outside while I get the car.'

James was slightly portly, wore glasses, and was about thirty-five.

'I teach chemistry,' he said. 'Your aunt has been very kind to me. She is quite a character, you know. Well liked in the town. A pity about the unfortunate affair of the rabbits.'

He stood to attention by the side of the lane awaiting Aunt Sarah's car. I did likewise, fixing my eye on the wall opposite.

'Gerbils,' I corrected him.

'No, no,' replied James sotto voce. 'It was Nganhong who ate May Sneadon's baby rabbits. I happen to know her husband. He is a school gardener. Why did you say gerbils?' he asked, seeing me squirm.

'Nothing,' I said, tight-lipped.

'I see,' he said. 'In fact, I am afraid to ask more.'

Just then Aunt Sarah, the picture of innocence, turned up.

'Cats are carnivores,' I said, defending my aunt.

'Quite, quite,' James affirmed. 'Less said the better, no point upsetting anyone. No point at all. Doesn't bother me. Do you mind if I sit in the front?'

'No, on you go,' I jumped in the back. 'What is planned. Are we all going to be swimming three lengths?'

'Wait and see,' was the enigmatic reply.

'I am concerned, Sarah, that you have got me some trunks that fit and are not rude in texture, shape or form.' James was deliberately pompous.

Aunt Sarah sniggered. 'No, they are fine. I guarantee.'

We arrived at the pool. Aunt Sarah insisted on paying for us. James and I padded through to the changing rooms. We walked along in style reminiscent of Taliban at Camp X-ray out for a five-minute breather. There was little enthusiasm to be seen in our gait.

'Better get over with it,' said James. 'Your aunt usually has some good outings, but I think this may be one too far.' His trunks were neat and did their best to contain with decorum his pale paunch. Mine were a little of the same.

'Good, good, you two look fine,' said Aunt Sarah, greeting us. She was in a one-piece green bathing suit, and was, I could now see, very fit. James and I looked at each other. We moved round the pool after Sarah. 'We are just going to go down these flumes, here.' She pointed to a side entrance. In we went. 'Now I know both of you are okay for health,' she said as we passed the signs asking us if we ever fainted, had high blood pressure or were unfit.

'*How come?*' demanded James and myself in unison.

'Oh,' replied Aunt Sarah, handing me the soft foam carpet I was to lie on. 'I phoned Jill last night when you had gone to bed. She knew you would probably forget to phone and I asked her then. She says good luck, by the way. And for you, James, the school medic told me.'

'He shouldn't have!' expostulated James.

'I only asked him if any teacher in the Chemistry Department had – what does it say here? – high blood pressure, giddiness, strokes et cetera. He told me you were all fit, even for a parachute jump. So I took that as a yes. Come on, James. Besides, I know that shape hides a committed bicyclist and a serious chemist.' Up she went, with teenagers dodging around her.

'A cyclist, maybe, but not a someone slightly crazed,' mumbled James, following. We arrived at the first level. Aunt Sarah suggested we start there. She just popped into the hole and left James and myself staring.

'When it goes green, you go!' commanded the assistant.

James disappeared. Then I lay down on my mat. A little frisson of excitement came as I watched the red light and then pushed off with the green. Almost immediately there was a sudden stomach-losing drop. I remembered my cream cakes earlier in the morning and swallowed hard to keep them down. But there was no time for any more thought as I braced myself against some truly frightening sudden bends followed by a whirl of light and a great splash as I exited.

'Okay, okay, Aunt Sarah, it is good fun!' I admitted, as I

hauled myself out with a slight belch. The cream cakes had finally gone away down.

'I think it's great,' enthused James. His face was shining in spite of his wet hair and myopic stare. He looked like someone who is full of the joy of a recent conversion and baptism. He strode for the stairs with a purpose and smile. Aunt Sarah gave me a sly wink and followed. In the next few minutes we tried nearly all the flumes as happy as any teenagers. Then we wondered about the last one. It was the highest and the most breathtaking. It had a nickname: 'Voodoo 2'.

'I will need a witness,' explained James. 'No one in my classes will believe I did this unless you two come.'

Up we all went. The overseer examined each of us carefully. He prodded at James.

'You okay for this, sir? It's quite a ride. Read the medical notices?'

'He is okay. I am in charge of him,' said Aunt Sarah. The overseer looked at her well-toned body, nodded and let James on.

James went first, Sarah next. I had to wait an age. I wondered if something had gone wrong. I saw the overseer speak into the mike.

'You're clear to go at the next green,' he said. 'You must hold onto the mat and relax.'

It went green and I gingerly pushed myself forward. I was not going to rush this one. The first slope pulled me down a rapid slide and at the end it suddenly rose up. The white mat and I took off up in the air and then crashed into a little pool. This pool quickly sucked me toward a large plughole. Through the plughole and down to the left the flume curved. Then another sudden rush down, with the flume walls changing colours, and just as I thought I was going too fast the flume spiralled three times causing my whole body to become briefly fixed upside down on the roof of the flume three times. I screamed. A few very fast curves came next. A straight was followed by a loop-the-loop with water everywhere. Then I went through three walls of water jetting down from the roof. Next a kaleidoscope of lights shining through the walls. This was followed by a series of chicanes, quick left-right turns which knocked my head against the side walls. A precipitous drop came next, followed by a steep slope that rose up suddenly. The end of the flume rose up and I was catapulted high up above the receiving pool. I landed in a heap with a great splash. I made my way to the side.

'Okay, sir?' enquired the assistant

'Yeah, fine,' I replied, still trying to come to terms with what I had just gone through.

'You can collect your badge there.' He pointed to a board were a set of simple gold-coloured badges lay. I saw Aunt Sarah. She smiled. James was still looking beatific.

'I lost my mat at the bottom third,' said Aunt Sarah. 'A little bruise. It is nothing; we had to wait for my mat. He was very kind, the assistant. He said it happens with about one in four. Once more?'

'I am happy to watch. But I will keep anyone company who is needing.' I could see that James was now hooked on it.

'Well, I have succeeded,' said Sarah as we mounted the stairs again. We let her carry on. 'Neither of you are thinking about work now are you?'

'*Oh, we're not thinking about work!*' James and I shouted. Then like two urchins, we raced each other up the final stairs. The assistant smiled as he sent us down. This time we all arrived without mishap. We agreed it was time to go to the match. I heard James speaking to himself about how he could now die happy, and I smiled to myself.

Out in the car park the cold air hit us and so we hurried to St James's Park. The rest of the day passed in a whirl of entertainment and fun. There were only two other BP executives in the box. Both knew Aunt Sarah, and they determined to entertain us as if the company's reputation depended on it. Southampton scored in under two minutes but then the Magpies came back and ran out eventual winners 2–1.

At the final whistle Aunt Sarah was jumping up and down. Then she guided everyone, including the BP men, to a Chinese restaurant she knew. She explained that although the décor was not as fine as others we would get genuine Chinese food. Volleys of Mandarin shot out from her and the restaurateur when we arrived. We were treated like royalty; I was pleased for Aunt

Sarah, as I could see the BP men, who were well-seasoned travellers, were enjoying their meal enormously. The BP men insisted we go for 'at least one pint' in a genuine Geordie pub. After more than one pint, Aunt Sarah, still enjoying herself enormously, said time was up. We said goodbye to the men from BP. James and I lay comatose in the back of Aunt Sarah's car as we went home. I glimpsed her using a mobile phone. Then we stopped outside a house in Norbury. James woke up, recognised his house, and with profuse thanks tumbled out.

In a comfortable silence Aunt Sarah and I went back to her home. She had taught me that the mark of good friends was that silences are not uncomfortable.

'Bed, I think,' she said,

'I agree,' was my reply. 'That was a terrific time.'

'I will wake you tomorrow, Richard, night,'

'G'night,' I responded. In a contented daze, I negotiated the stairs and made it to bed.

Chapter Six

I always love to begin a journey on Sundays, because I shall have the prayers of the church, to preserve all that travel.

Jonathan Swift, 1667–1745

The tapping on the door awoke me.

'Richard, I'm going to Communion in twenty-five minutes. Are you able?'

'Yes, sure. Come in,' I croaked. Aunt Sarah came in carrying a mug of tea. She communicated in many different ways.

'This is for you. The service starts at eight. We're okay if we leave by ten to.'

I took the proffered mug and heaved myself up. Before I could say anything Aunt Sarah was gone. It would have to be a quick cup. Still, it was refreshing. Opening my suitcase I found Jill had packed a suit. Funny how women think of almost everything, I mused. I cleaned myself up and headed downstairs.

Aunt Sarah was below, waiting. She wore a dark coat. She had no make-up. Like my mother, she was a little old school and preferred to go to Communion on an empty stomach and with little or no bending to vanity. We walked in short clipped steps to the church. The town was silent. One or two equally dark-clothed people were walking to the church. Inside we were handed the flimsy Cambridge blue booklets. We found ourselves a pew halfway up on the right. It was a quiet, reverent service with no hymns and a short homily. Both of us preferred this form of service. I felt no one should speak for more than seven minutes: few nowadays could attend anything longer. Aunt Sarah admitted to enjoying loud worship, but paradoxically she felt the need for forgiveness and quiet reflection as more important. She also had a theory that there was nothing more nauseous than being part of some loud, insincere form of praise. I suspected this was a very English trait she had assimilated. On the way down from the altar after receiving Communion I almost bumped into James. He smiled and attempted to both recognise and ignore me at the same moment. I wondered if he had been guiding my Aunt Sarah through the foibles of the English.

At the end of the service we said our goodbyes to those we new. I nodded to Leasden, whom I saw helping an old lady to her car. Then we headed back.

'Cook day off, Sunday day off,' Aunt Sarah said, mimicking a poor Chinese attempt to speak English. She saw my look of surprise and pointed to the hotel opposite, The Last Redoubt.

'TLR!' To my surprise she knew the boys' nickname for the hotel. 'TLC at TLR from mater and pater' was the standard quote of us spoilt teenagers. We always guided our parents toward this hotel, famous for the quality and size of its table.

'Are you treating me like a schoolboy?' I asked suspiciously.

'No, no,' she remarked. 'It just has the best-cooked breakfast. Come on. I am fed up with cooking, even for you.'

It was a baroque-style room. Red carpets and ornate gold fittings predominated. The waiters were spotty youngsters but the food they brought was impeccable.

'Now all we need is some Sunday newspapers and some time to digest all that. Don't you agree?'

I nodded in acquiescence. In ten minutes we were back in the sitting room, lounging in chairs and idly flipping through three Sunday papers and exchanging comments. Wooihfung and Nganhong were desperately trying to get our attention. Aunt Sarah got up to put them out the back door. I heard a muffled exclamation and went to find her. Standing on the doorway, I saw her look down at her feet. Three dead mice lay on the doorstep: offerings on an altar made by the cats. The cats walked this way and that, mewing as if to ask for appreciation of their night's work. Aunt Sarah held her hand to her mouth.

'They really are terrible,' she said. A small tear came in her eye. 'Well, I had better just get rid of them.' She put on some washing up gloves and went out to the garden with a trowel carrying the mice. We stopped by a small bush.

83

'This is the place I put them all. I have lost count completely. James has an awful sense of humour and has asked if he can write to the Commonwealth Graves Commission to have this plot registered.' She sighed. 'In fact, he said it was getting like some atrocity from the Balkans. But then when he said that about the atrocity your Classics Master, Leasden, reprimanded him for bad taste. Schoolboys, schoolboys.' She finished the burial of the mice, stood up, took off her gloves, brushed her skirt and headed for the door.

Once inside and back with the Sunday papers her good humour returned. The phone rang. Aunt Sarah went down to the hall to answer it. She came back.

'A walk on the fells?' She cocked her head. 'I said we might go. But I didn't commit us, only if you want to.' I glanced outside; the sun was offering to break through.

'Yes, but I haven't got any boots. Wait – I have my wellies in the car. Good idea, some exercise. We don't have to go right now, do we? Besides, who is going?'

'Oh, no. Three-quarters of an hour. James said he had to arrange the others. I have some other boots if you care to try.' Those must be my uncle's boots, I thought. She has kept hold of them all these years.

'Fair enough, sounds good to me.'

Aunt Sarah disappeared down the hallway to reply. We leafed through the rest of the papers and then got ready. A white van appeared. James was at the wheel. He seemed particularly cheery.

'I am on the wagon today. Climb aboard. Sarah, Richard, you know Claude.' I saw him point to Leasden; he nodded. I returned his nod. 'And Damian, his wife, Justine, and Geoffrey. No, not everyone has a connection with the college. Make yourselves acquainted.'

We sat at the rear obeying his instructions. Damian and Justine were not at the college but they did have an educational background. Damian was an Old Etonian who taught art at the grammar school... 'For kicks,' he explained. His wife Justine was enjoying a day off. Her mother-in-law had taken charge of their two children. Geoffrey was a traffic warden. It seemed stupid to tell him that I had never met a traffic warden before. I mentioned this as a reflex comment and immediately the others were engulfed in laughter. I did not understand until he said something along the lines of, 'Some us don't return to the Planet Zog every night but fraternise with the Earthlings.' James screamed with delight when he heard this. I had fallen for the one social gaffe they most enjoyed. Leasden and Aunt Sarah merely smiled, shaking their heads.

The van headed for the Northumbrian hills. The countryside was speckled with dark and light as the sun broke through the patchy clouds. Although the fields were similar to Scotland, being divided by stone dykes with a large number of livestock hidden in them, it was not the same. The hills were more rolling and windswept, there was less relief and the sky was mundane in comparison.

James parked the van midway down a valley. On either side hills rose above us. On one side was a remarkable sight. A series of standing stones in two rows twenty yards apart walked up the slope to a summit about two thousand feet above us.

'Amazing!' I exclaimed.

'Yes, it is very impressive, if you have a historical or classical bent,' explained James. 'These are standing stones which lead all the way up to the hill fort at the top.' He pointed to an extra rise at the top. 'Undoubtedly built by the Ancient Britons; the Romans hardly touched this site. They found it a bit- spooky. It smelt to them of spirits. At the top is a vitrified fort. The stones of the walls are fused together. Now, the heat required to do this is incredible. In fact, no one can work out how they managed to produce such a furnace heat there.' We all gazed in silence.

'More importantly, just the other side of this hill is a road, and on it is one of the highest pubs in Britain. So that is our mission: except for Geoffrey, who has kindly volunteered to drive the van there to save our limbs.' We all turned to Geoffrey in a mixture of thankfulness and envy.

'Warm up a little before we go. Any questions?'

Damian's hand shot up. 'You have been in the army, haven't you James? You never told me that.' James looked bemused and shook his head. Leasden filled in.

'No, he has not been in the army, but I gather he has to assist with the school cadet force.'

We all checked our boots and started the climb up. Almost as if it had been planned Aunt Sarah and Justine started walking together, chatting about their children. James and Damian started talking about hills they had climbed. This left Leasden and me together. We had little to talk about. I could see by the way he walked with sure, measured steps he had walked the fells before. We mounted the slope midway between the two rows of standing stones. Every few hundred yards or so we would stop for half a minute or two, catch our breath and turn and admire the scenery. The top was not so obvious due to the angle of the slope.

Mists or clouds suddenly came down upon us. James halted us and gathered us near the left row of standing stones. He checked his bearing on the compass and then instructed us to climb up the left-hand stones but on the right side of them. If we strayed in any direction we would then come across one line of standing stones. The clouds cleared every now and then with the result that for a brief moment the sun beat down upon us. All we could see were clouds surrounding us. A view of any distance was impossible. Then thin clouds descended and we would be walking in an eerie atmosphere, with the bright cloud not quite clearing yet allowing the sun to give us light. We could see why the Romans regarded this area as ghostlike. Leasden stopped as some particularly thick cloud swirled around us. He looked up at the bodies mounting the slope ahead of us in a file near the standing stones.

'Extraordinary – that reminds me of something,' he observed.

I joined him and looked at the shapes in the yards ahead of me. The standing stones and the walkers all appeared similar. Only the movement of the walkers distinguished them. I expected Leasden to comment on some past Greek battle. Instead he said, 'That's it. Washington!'

'Washington…' I sounded doubtful.

'Yes, it is like the US Veterans' memorial to the Korean War at Washington. You see these shadowy figures walking though the mists. It is very moving. The standing stones and those figures are very similar. Men patrolling though the mist with care and power. Have you been to Washington?'

'No.'

'Oh, well. You wouldn't see what I mean. In fact you probably think I am being an awful snob. But the likeness is uncanny. We had better go on.'

On we strode to catch up. As we gained height the clouds came down on us with greater frequency. Just before we reached the fort we had a view of it a hundred yards above us. It was one solid dark band with no distinguishing features. Then came thick mist. The first we knew of the fort was finding an enormous number of small boulders all glued to each other. We paused. It was obvious that an extremely fierce fire could be the only cause for the fusion of the stones. We scrambled up the slope over these stones and reached the top. Fortunately the clouds cleared a little and we gazed around at the hill fort. The mound of fused blocks formed a large oval wall, which could hold half a football pitch. There was no view of the surrounding countryside. We descended carefully down to the bottom and found it very quiet. The walls cut out the sound. Clouds scudded over us. James handed out a small snack to everyone, took a compass bearing and pointed us out over the wall on the other side. Up and over it we went. Again, there was no view to admire. James checked his bearing and we followed him.

Soon he found the stream he was looking for. It had a path beside it through the heather. This side of the hill was some form of moor. The clouds cleared and we could see a road not too far down below and one white-walled building. That was our destination. As we came within site of our lunch, our walking accelerated. In no time we found ourselves in the pub. A sign asked us to remove boots, if muddy, which most of us did. In we went to find Geoffrey propping up the bar.

'Good timing!' he said. 'I have just finished my soft drink.' We all felt a great sense of relaxation with all the hard work over. Leasden bought everyone the first round. A ploughman's lunch to each of us followed from James and Geoffrey.

'We put you through the purgatory, so eat up, and no complaints,' said Geoffrey. 'You can't say traffic wardens are all bad now,' he added.

Leasden asked me whether I was staying the night. I said no, I had to leave for the North.

'Oh. Are you going through Edinburgh?' he asked

'Yes, I usually do. I find it quicker.'

'Any chance you can give me a lift? I could drive myself but it would be useful for me.'

I felt a kick and saw a look from my aunt. 'Yes, why not?' I said, feeling the opposite. It was as if I had joined the ranks of those perennial liars, the diplomats.

'Fine! Well, if your car is covered for two drivers, I can drive the first bit to Edinburgh, and you can now have another pint. It will have worn off by the time you take over.'

'Yes, why not?' I repeated the words like an immigrant who has just found a use for a newly-learnt English phrase. Leasden gave me a queer look and I smile reassuringly back at him. The drink as usual relieved me of my fluttering worries. What was I to say to him on the car journey? The rest of the afternoon flowed on in a benign haze, so that my next concentrated moment found me opposite Aunt Sarah's house, my case in the car and about to head back home.

'Thanks for a wonderful weekend, Aunt. Took me away from everything.' I kissed her on the cheek.

'Well, I enjoyed it too,' she returned. 'Now be good.' She winked as Leasden appeared and walked up. 'Don't worry, you will be fine after Edinburgh,' she whispered.

Leasden soon had a grasp of the car and we shot off. I waved to Aunt Sarah. Wooihfung and Nganhong were just two white blobs on the inside window sill.

'There's no need for you to chat,' said Leasden. 'In fact, if you do not mind me being a little abrupt, I would take a kip if I were you. I know the road north of Edinburgh. It would be better for you if you took a wink or two now.' I couldn't beat this sensible suggestion.

Leasden woke me just short of Edinburgh.

'You don't think I am mad?' he asked.

'No,' I replied, 'not for a Classics Master,' and we both laughed.

'Well, bearing in mind that we are about to come to the Athens of the North, listen to this.'

He turned up the volume of the CD player. It dawned on me that he had been quietly listening to Wagner. I recognised the last part of the *Tannhäuser* overture. High ahead of us we could see the lights of the city reflected in the sky. They were bordered at the base by the dark Pentland Hills rising up. As we climbed the hills the music hinted at the advent of something new. A terrific crash broke out from the CD player when we emerged from the gloom of the hills at the summit and found the shining lights of the city of Edinburgh in front of us. We descended to the city over the switchback curves, accompanied by the descending repetitive notes of *Tannhäuser*. It occurred to me that Leasden was a romantic of the first order. He stopped just beyond the first roundabout.

'This is where I leave you. You can manage?' He stared at me.

'Are you sure?' I wondered if he was being realistic.

'Yes, I can get a taxi from here. No need for you to come into town any further. The traffic is poor. Leaving Edinburgh, you need *Lohengrin*, Prelude to Act Three. It is on track four. You can keep the CD, or if you feel uncomfortable post it to your aunt she will give to me via James.' He slammed the door and was gone, raising his hand hailing a taxi. I shook my head, changed to track four and crossed the Forth Road Bridge with the *Lohengrin* driving me Northward.

At home all were in bed. Jill shouted down, 'Is that you, Richard?'

'It had better be!' I quipped. 'Anything new?'

'Oh, nothing… your aunt phoned. She said she hoped you didn't mind taking – what is his name? – Leaser. It is just she didn't want you to appear rude. I agreed that was important; we then had a long chat.'

'I bet you did. Leasden, not Leaser. He is well. I must admit I did see another side to him. But still I am not a fan of his.'

'Aunt Sarah didn't, I am sure, want you to be a fan, just considerate. Anyway, come to bed. It's late. You can tell me all about it tomorrow.'

Chapter Seven

Utinam per unam diem essemus bene conversati in hoc mundo –
O that we had spent but one day in this world thoroughly
well!

Thomas a Kempis, 1380–1471

'Your sweater is inside out,' Emma informed me. I put my hand
round the back of my neck and found the label to confirm her
observation; the children had gone without much fuss at breakfast
time, but after a good weekend I had not got it all together yet.

'Tea, please,' I replied.

Emma got up. In the next room she shouted to me from
beside the kettle. 'Did you have a good weekend?'

'Yes, thanks. I saw my aunt. Caught up with her. Climbed a
hill, saw a football match and even went down a flume.'

'Sounds good,' said Emma, returning. 'Not much happened
here. At least, nothing too untoward.' She started opening some
of the mail and Neil came in.

'Ah, Richard! Good weekend?' He could see in my rosy
cheeks the face of someone who has relaxed for a day or two. This
always contrasts with the pallor of the person who has just
completed a weekend on duty.

'Yes thanks, Neil. All well?' I asked.

'Perhaps,' said Neil. 'Your friend Mrs Brown, Lochhead Farm
has—'

'Not my friend, Neil,' I cut in on him. 'I warned you before
have nothing to do with that woman. She is dangerous. I told you
what she has done with other practices and to me. That was when
I was a new graduate well over ten years ago.'

She had on that occasion watched me take the temperature of
a calf and then chastised me for not believing her own reading of
the temperature taken from the same calf half an hour before. 'I

can take a temperature!' she had shouted at me from a yard away. 'I have done a course.' I did not disbelieve her but had merely gone through my routine. From then on anything I did on Mrs Brown's farm had to be justified to the last minute reason. On another occasion she had reported a young lady vet to the Royal College for using an antibiotic that saved a horse's life. The antibiotic had not been licensed for use with horses, as Mrs Brown had discovered on reading the label. She refused to pay the bill and lodged a formal complaint.

'Neil, I hope you have not agreed to treat anything of hers...' I rambled on.

'Not quite...' Neil tried to explain.

'It won't be worth the heartache and worry. She is so two-faced. Butter wouldn't melt when she is here in this waiting room or chatting to the senior partner. But once your back is turned – watch out!' I was determined Neil got the message. 'I know this from some of the local folk my wife knows. Jill gets all the gossip. This could be a bad start to the week, you know. What have you done for her? You haven't signed some document, or something? She once tried to get Phil to sign and date a vaccination card for a different date of the vaccination, you know.' I again emphasised my points. Practice had enough stress without taking on litigious clients.

'Your friend, Mrs Brown...'

'Not my *friend*, Neil; *acquaintance*, perhaps,' I declared quietly.

'Your *friend*, Richard,' Neil batted on, 'has just been found dead suddenly for no obvious reason.'

'Oh... ohh.' I paused, taken aback. 'Ah well, I have nothing to say.'

'Your previous comments?' Neil hunted for an explanation from me. I was silent. He smirked. 'I will take that as a recantation.'

'I am sure we have got some work to do,' I said to change the subject.

'Mrs Sneyd for you, Richard.' Emma handed me the card. Mrs Sneyd and I entered the consulting room.

'What can I do to help?' I asked. After Neil's lesson I was prepared to be a saint for anyone.

'It's his glands – I think. He keeps on rubbing his bottom and squeaking,' she said, dumping the irate Westie on the table. Normally a case of anal glands first thing Monday morning dulls my bonhomie. But now I was in an angelic mood.

'Oh, I am sure we can sort that out.' I looked at the record card. The anal glands had been emptied six months before. He was only two years old. I grabbed various accroutments – cotton wool, gloves, lubricating fluid – and asked her to hold him tight.

'It is just the dog equivalent of skunk glands, and they get blocked occasionally,' I explained, as I squeezed the glands one by one and emptied their foetid contents on to the cotton wool. 'When I first qualified there were one or two brave old boys who did this job with their bare hands.'

Mrs Sneyd looked at me in disbelief. The Westie had braced himself; he bared his teeth in a forced grin and growled at me. I didn't blame him; it must have been pretty uncomfortable. He next received an injection. Then I explained some of the ins and outs of the condition to Mrs Sneyd and the importance of diet. If he kept on coming back with the same problem we might have to agree to remove the glands with a surgical operation.

As soon as I handed in one record card June gave me another. 'Mrs Gauld and Sooty,' she informed me. Mrs Gauld followed me in. She was dressed for the office and had probably taken an hour off to bring her pet in.

'I wasn't going to come until this evening. But he is so lame that I couldn't bear leaving him. I wonder if he has broken something,' she explained and immediately opened the cage door. Sooty, a black and white cat, poked his head out to take one look round and then went back. Put yourself in his position, and that is an intelligent move, I thought.

'Sooty, come out, please.' The tone of voice often gives a clue as to how close and genuine the relationship is. She was obviously very attached to her cat. Sooty, deep inside the solid plastic cage, mewed plaintively. He was torn between the two. Reason told him to stay in the safe cage; emotion told him to go and speak to his mistress. Once again, Mrs Gauld pleaded with him. 'Come on out, it will be okay.' He mewed back in return. They both began to implore each other with a duet of human beseeching and cat mewing. The scene was becoming operatic, both in its emotion and otherworldly drama.

'Here, let me help. This is, after all, where their mothers grab them.'

I put my hand carefully in the cage, grabbed Sooty's scruff and pulled the cage away from him. It was not unlike pulling a hermit crab out of his shell. I shut the door of the cage, to which Sooty had immediately attempted a retreat. He was not putting much weight on his right front foot. I peered at it and noticed a small area around the wrist. Here, the hair was clumped together. Mrs Gauld wore a concerned frown.

'I think I will ask June to help me,' I said. 'There may be an abscess on the wrist from a cat bite. It may be sore to examine.'

Cat bite abscesses were routine, but many a slip could be made. I opened the door and called June in. June has her own cats, which she dotes on, yet she is also firm when required. I appreciated her sure touch. She held Sooty firmly while I touched the swollen wrist.

'I am going to remove this scab. It may be a little sore but hopefully it may allow some drainage and mess come out.' I pulled at the scab. Sooty wriggled. June held firm and muttered a sweet nothing to the cat. Sure enough, a dribble of green-yellow pus and dark red blood came out from the spot where I had removed the scab.

'Oh!' said Mrs Gauld. 'How horrible! At least I know it is not broken.'

June wrinkled her nose at the sight and smell. I quickly cleaned up the area and gave an injection. Then June dispensed some pills, with instructions on how to keep the wound open for a day or two to allow drainage.

'We will see you on Friday, by which time I am sure it will be fine. If you are at all worried do call us. But normally this clears up fine.' This was my parting shot, and off went Mrs Gauld for another day in the office.

'Could you answer the phone, Richard?' asked Emma as I went back in the office. 'June is down the back checking some drugs.'

I picked up the phone and rehearsed the usual phrase.

'Inverden Veterinary Centre.' There was silence at the other end of the phone and then a voice with a distant, hollow timbre spoke.

'Can I speak to someone?' I thought for a second of the implications of the question.

'Yes, you can.' Another silence.

'I want to speak to a vet, not a nurse,' the voice informed me.

'Well, I am a vet. Richard Jones. How can I help you?' I tried to clarify matters.

'Can I speak to the lady vet – Anne. No offence to you,' continued the voice still in a deep hollow tone.

'No offence to me, but I'm afraid she is consulting now. If I can't help you, could you leave your name, phone number, address and the query and I am sure she will phone back?'

Anne was our veterinary assistant who made up the third part of our three-vet practice. She was a very competent vet and Neil, in spite of his preference for male vets had employed her purely on merit. Since then his trust in her abilities had been well rewarded, and as a result we expected to make her a partner soon.

'That is a good idea, I will phone back later.' Click went the phone. I put it down with a bemused expression.

'Problems?' prompted June.

'Oh, I think I will leave odd callers like that to you professionals, June. That one was a bit beyond me.'

'I think it must be the moon or something that's bringing them out this week,' volunteered June. 'I have had quite a few this morning already while you have been consulting. Mrs Dear phoned to ask for the time of her appointment. She couldn't remember it, and the dog had just eaten the appointment card. Then I had to phone Mrs Macrae to remind her to bring in her cat. When I phoned and asked to speak to Mrs Macrae the voice at the other end said, "Maybe you can. Who is it?" I said it was the vets and then the voice said, "Then in that case I *am* Mrs Macrae. What is it all about?" So I told her she needed to bring Coco in for his injection. She said fine she would come in at two p.m. Then Mrs Smith came in to pay for her dog food and I asked her how she was and she said, "Not too good, I'm afraid; I have just discharged myself after taking an overdose".'

'Goodness, will she be okay?' I asked.

'I think so. She was accompanied here by a relative who was keeping very close to her. It is not Mrs Smith from Hale Farm, a different one. Anyway, here is one more for you – Mrs Whyte. She can't get a pill down Bunty, so she has come to the professionals.'

I neglected to say that one of my cats had not had a pill for two years because it would maul me, and in the end I had resorted to other powders and pour-ons to deal with said cat.

'Right. Let's see what I can do. Mrs Whyte, please come with me.'

'I feel so stupid that I can't do this but she is the very devil, you know. She did this to me yesterday,' she said. Mrs Whyte bared her arm up to her elbow and revealed red lines at least three inches long where the cat had 'cluked' her.

'You did see a doctor about that, didn't you?' I asked.

'Practice nurse… she gave me a clean-up and some antibiotics after she spoke to a doctor.'

'Fair enough. Let us see your tiger.' I opened the cat-cage door and removed the cat. She was small, black, and maintained a wicked expression. I had seen quite a few like that before. Although they were small they possessed the capability to turn into a ball of fire and strike like a cobra.

'Doesn't look much, does she?' commented Mrs Whyte, almost in embarrassment.

'Don't you worry, I can quite believe you. She may well be a handful. We will try and put a pill down her now. Then we will discuss other options which are more practical for you.' I went to the door. 'June, can you come here, please? I need your skill at restraint.'

Mrs Whyte stepped back while June entered and came forward, mimicking the smooth movement of a judo black belt.

'Don't trust little Bunty an inch, June,' I advised her, as I found a worming pill.

June surrounded the cat, holding her scruff and two elbows. I held the head, at which point Bunty extended all her claws and hissed malevolently. Thanks to June's hold, Bunty's wide-open claws swathed through the air but caught nothing. With one finger I pulled Bunty's lower jaw down, and with another I quickly pushed a pill down to the rear of her pharynx. Bunty's eyeballs bulged up in a surprised look and she swallowed. It was all over. With our usual teamwork we immediately released her. Bunty sat still, immobilised with surprise.

'Thank you, June. I doubt, Mrs Whyte, that we can always treat her. One day she may better us, even if we use a pill popper for pushing the pill right down. Outside I'll show you some other way to do this with powders and pour-on droplets.'

'I think that might be better. It would be less stressful for her – and for me, come to that.' We all trooped out of the room.

'I have got one more for you before tea and some calls for you to do,' said Emma. 'Mrs Paterson and Jake. You asked them to come back for a final blood sample.'

'Oh yes, this'll be interesting.'

In practice the main body of small animal work is routine to the point of boredom. It can be hard to inject enthusiasm in to such a mundane workload. Then something like Jake turns up. He had come into the surgery very ill – and for no apparent reason. His main presenting signs were odd coloured urine, poor appetite, a fever and pale gums. My gut feeling was that he was suffering from a disease where the body, through its immune system of antibodies and white cells, attacks itself. In this case it attacks its own red blood cells, hence the conditions name autoimmune haemolytic anaemia (AHA). Even though it is an uncommon condition there are many different types of AHA. Fortunately the treatments are very similar. We had started the treatment immediately and blood sampled him to see if we could confirm the condition. Luckily for us, he had responded quickly to the steroids we gave him and the blood samples were consistent with the diagnosis. Among other things they showed he had severe anaemia. I had also put a little blood on a microscope slide. The blood had formed clumps which were also suggestive of AHA. Our second blood sample a fortnight later had showed that he was returning to normal and now we were taking a third one. We hoped to find a normal result.

'Come in, come in,' I said to Mr and Mrs Paterson. Jake, the cocker spaniel, came bouncing in.

'He is completely different from a month ago,' said Mrs Paterson enthusiastically. The dog obviously meant a lot to these pensioners.

'Well, I think we have been quite lucky. We got a good response to the treatment: no relapses and his blood picture is returning to normal. He is on two pills a day, isn't he?' They nodded. 'Well, we may reduce that a little yet. Anyway, we will take this step by step. So Emma and I will just take this sample now and send it off to check.'

I had a look at Jake. He was fine. Though it was good to see him I had to confess I got a greater kick out of seeing him from a distance being taken out for a walk in the streets of Inverden. There was another dog in the town with the same condition. Both were treasured pets and would not be walking the streets if a vet hadn't treated them. It was fun to see them from far away and think how lucky they were to be alive.

Jake wriggled a little but soon we had what we wanted. I held up the blood tube while Emma put the treasured canine down on the ground, and off he walked back to his owners, his stubby tail wiggling backwards and forwards furiously.

'I'll phone you tomorrow. But it does appear fine at the moment,' I said as they went on their way.

'Tea?' said Emma.

'Fine – what have you got for me?' I asked.

'Just two calls at the moment,' said June, examining the daybook. 'Mr Davidson, Millhill, and Mr Ratray, Nether Dags. Neither are urgent.' I finished my tea quickly.

'I'll go to Nether Dags first.'

I drove out past the cemetery on the edges of the town and over a bridge. Below by the river there were one or two townsfolk salmon fishing. They had rights to fish near the town. After the bridge I passed by some arable fields; glancing back across the fields I could make out the school clock tower surrounded by linden trees. Then the road disappeared into forestry land. The road was darker here and hid a series of dangerous concealed exits. Eventually it gave way to wide open fields dotted with few farms and divided by long rough stone dykes. Five miles out from Inverden, I turned off up a steep farm track full of loose stones.

Eventually I drove over a small bridge with a burn under it and up into the main court of the farm.

'A dry day so far,' I commented to Mr Ratray.

'Aye, it may hold dry yet.' He turned away toward a farm building and I followed him. We entered through a narrow doorway into the dark building. There was a long trough full of barley, and a wheelbarrow at one end. Mechanisation had not yet reached this part of the farm.

'What's worst with him?' I asked.

'I'm not very sure. He could have got too much barley. But then they have been on it for two months or more. Still, I thought you had better check this one, and I may have another.'

It often occurred in our world that the farmer would offer the opportunity to go the second mile. I wondered what GPs would make of it if at some point in the consultation the patient said, 'While you're here, I have another family member outside in the waiting room – I hoped you would have the time to see my relative now. After all, I pay my tax like anyone else.' The proposition was ridiculous, and yet we undertook this all the time. One good reason for this is that vets are often dealing with herd problems, and a good look at a second or third animal may well give clues as to what the underlying problem is on the farm. It also means more business to the vet practice, which is not financed in the same manner as the NHS.

'Is that your other one?' I asked, pointing to one stirk (yearling) which was lying down. The stirk rose slowly and wobbled away. It was as though he was drunk.

'Aye, that's the one,' concurred Mr Ratray. 'He looks a little worse for it.'

'Well, we had better check both. Can we get them into the crush if possible?'

'Aye. Give me a minute to set a couple of gates,'

Mr Ratray went to the other end of the court and set a gate leading to a crush. We coaxed one of the stirks along the wall to the crush, weeding out the ones we didn't want. The stirk was slow, slightly blown up and with a dull look to his head. If it was barley poisoning, or to give it another name, 'grain overload', then he would have quite a headache and feel pretty liverish. He halted halfway in the crush and we put our shoulders on his backside, pushed him forward, and trapped his head in the front of the crush. I stood back to get my thermometer out of my pocket. The stirk coughed and some very moist faeces flew past my left ear. Diarrhoea dribbled down his perineum.

'That is a good sign if he has eaten too much barley. He'll purge most of the excess away,' I observed. After a minute or two I read the temperature. It was up half a degree. The eye mucus membranes were very red, typical of the acidosis in the animal. The extra barley had fermented rapidly in the rumen, producing excess acid amongst other by-products. As a result of the chemical reaction water is drawn into the rumen, and this tends to dehydrate the rest of the animal. With my stethoscope I could hear odd gassy noises in the rumen, which was relatively immobile and full of gas and ingesta. The heart rate and breathing rate was slightly high. The poor beast was trying, among other things, to 'blow off' carbon dioxide in order to compensate for the extra acid. In biochemical terms this was pretty futile. I completed my examination.

'Well, farmers are right nineteen times out of twenty. I also think he has had too much barley. He is standing and his heart rate is not too fast. It's not too severe, so we'll just give him a dose of milk of magnesia over the throat, some B vitamins in the vein, and put him on hay and water for a few days. Start him up on barley very gently after that. Have you got a bottle I can use for drenching him with?'

'Aye,' said Mr Ratray, and off he went to find it. A few minutes later we met again at the crush and proceeded to treat him. Down went a litre and a half of milk of magnesia. It was very sticky. Then Mr Ratray put a halter on the stirk, raised the head up and I found the jugular vein and put forty millilitres of B vitamins into his blood system.

'That should do. Let's find the other.' We searched around for the other and soon had him in the crush too. He was much the same as the other except his nose was very dry and he had no diarrhoea.

'This one is a little worse than the other. You will have to give him another shot of B vitamins tomorrow. Anyway, see how he goes. If he's not offering to eat any hay tomorrow give me a shout. We can give him a drip, but I normally only do that if they can't stand.'

'Aye, aye.' Mr Ratray had seen many cases of barley poisoning and had a fair idea what to expect. We then discussed the presentation of the feed to the stirks and how it was possible if a mistake was made for one individual to eat much more than another. I cleaned my wellies and said my goodbyes.

'Vet Three to base,' I radioed in.

'Nothing new, Vet Three,' replied Emma.

'Okay, going on to Davidson.'

My car slithered down the stones of Mr Ratray's farm track and finally bounced onto the main road. Four more miles and on a relatively flat piece of countryside I found myself in the court of Mr Davidson.

'Pneumonia, I think. Two of them. But ye'll ken for certain,' was his opening remark.

'How old are they?' I asked.

'Oh, about two to three months. They're not bought in or anything. I gave them their injection of vitamin E and selenium at birth. But I must admit these few I haven't vaccinated or given a second vitamin injection. I was just waiting until I had a batch of five to do.'

The vaccine usually came in five-dose vials. We went into the building and moved some of the calves from the main group though a gap in some gates into the calf creep area where the cow cannot enter. Then we let back all the calves except the two we needed and we blocked off the escape hole. Next Mr Davidson grabbed one and pinned it to the wall. It coughed and showed remarkably quick breathing. The latter may have been due as much to the chase and fright as to any chest pathology. We handled it quickly. Checking its chest, joints, navel, temperature, ear, nose, throat, and lymph glands, I agreed it appeared to be a fairly straightforward bronchopneumonia. The list of causes was long. From a tray I had brought I selected three injections; an antibiotic; an anti-inflammatory medicine which went into the vein; and a vitamin injection. We then grabbed the other calf.

'Funny, his gums look pale,' I murmured. We looked closely

at him. His coat looked a bit rough. Peering closer I saw small dark objects on the skin around his shoulder blades. These were lice sucking blood from the calf.

'He's got lice as well as pneumonia. Unfortunately the good old days of effective louse powder have gone, so I will give him some Ivomec as well as the antibiotics and so on. You may have to put a pour-on on him as well.'

'Aye, I kept a goodly stock of that powder but it's all done now. It is funny how so many of the really good simple treatments have gone. You would have thought for calves it wouldn't make much difference to the beef eaten later. I remember calves almost white with the powder: it didn't poison them but, by God, it kept the lice away. You could use it for hens as well.'

Mr Davidson looked indignant. I decided not to carry on down that path much further. Some of the medicine legislation was bewildering when interpreted on the farm level.

'It is a bit early in the year for this type of condition but every now and then you get as surprise. Anyway, when you have time you could check some of others for lice.' I loaded up some syringes and treated the animal. We soon made our way to the tap to clean up and then I was back on the road.

'Vet Three to base,' I said, while I grabbed a piece of chocolate that was handy on the passenger seat.

'Ah, hello Richard. Can you go to Morden, Boghough?' replied Emma. 'He has a calf that keeps on blowing up. He thinks it might need a hole in its side or something. But you'll ken when you get there.' The farm was about twelve miles away, which was a fair detour. Emma has sixth sense, so she radioed again. 'Neil's been called to a calving and he wanted someone sooner rather than later as the calf is a little breathless.'

'Righto,' I said. Farmers' assessment of urgency is usually pretty good. Once, however, I had a memorable case where a farmer called me out to a calf 'with a touch of flu'. I had had nothing better to do so I had gone out immediately. When I arrived I found the calf with fulminating pneumonia and breathing its last. Ever since then, if that same farmer ever said anything had a 'touch' of something we raced out to see it.

My drive took me through many wooded areas and hills which Scotland is rightly famous for. Stone dykes ran over steep low hills which gave a sense of relief to the countryside. Many of these dykes were in poor repair with bracken or weeds growing on them. On occasion the dyke had fallen into complete disrepair, and so a barbed-wire fence could be found hard against the stones. Now and then I could see a solid country house or farm standing off the road. The roads were empty relative to the Home Counties in England and a delight to drive down on a day like this. After twenty-five minutes I had reached the farm. I parked my car on the left side of a muddy court that sloped up on either side. A small trickle of water, hardly a stream, flowed from further up the hill through the court along the dip in the middle. The door of the car swung open as I released the catch. I tipped myself out of the car and down to the centre of the court.

Mr Morden appeared in his customary oilskins. The weather was often poor near his farm, and half the ground was up on a steep slope more reminiscent of the Andes than Scotland. I looked out away from the farm buildings to the river far below and the bothies on the other side of the valley. A track led to each one and then disappeared off to join the nearest metalled road. Various stone dykes divided the fields on that side. There was no bridge across. If you needed to drive to those fields you had to negotiate a long detour. I had arrived once to be told by Mr Morden that the animal was in a field on the other side. I could either chance some well-spaced stepping-stones or drive the long way round. I chose the long way; that way I had all my drugs to hand.

'It is in the building here,' intimated Mr Morden.

I followed him up a dark corridor past three collies, all tied up. I faced each one in turn.

'They're not too bad. It's this one you want to watch: just wait here.'

Mr Morden went up to a fourth collie tied up at the top of the corridor. He held onto its collar firmly. The dog twisted and lunged in my direction. I nipped into the byre. Mr Morden followed. In a small closed off space were four calves. He was keeping them on one dairy cow; she was tied up at the far end. Three calves were fine, but one was blown up and had a stomach as tight as a drum.

'Does it tend to blow up just after it has taken the milk?' I queried.

'Na,' replied Mr Morden. 'If anything, it goes down a bit then.'

'Oh. Has it ever had pneumonia?'

'Aye, I have had to treat it twice before it did this carry-on with blowing up. It's lost a bit of condition, as you can see.' Mr Morden indicated that it was not his favourite animal. 'I have been putting a soft tube down to release the gas and that works fine. But I'm feart to find it dead one morning blown up like a ruddy great balloon.'

I nodded. We took hold of the calf. I noticed it had a nasal discharge and a bit of a cough. Its temperature was normal. The lungs sounded as though there was a suggestion of pneumonia.

'I think it has chronic pneumonia,' I informed him. 'They often have a normal temperature, and amongst other things the glands in the chest swell and act as a valve stopping the gas getting out.'

'Ah, my brither had a couple like that. I mind him telling me a few years ago.' Mr Morden shook his head.

'And what happened?' I followed up.

'Och, one lived, one died. They both got holes in the side and were drugged for a whiley.' he stared directly at me.

'That is about it,' I agreed. 'Still, we have to do it; otherwise you're right – you will find it dead one day. I think I can give you better odds than fifty-fifty, though. Can you help me back to the car?' I pointed my chin at his biting collie who had been listening in by the door.

'Sure, you just get your stuff. Do you need any water?' he said as he held the dog tight.

'Yes, that will be fine.'

Five minutes later we had the calf haltered and held tight against the panel of a byre divider. A naked bulb gave us some light. I clipped up the flank opposite to the rumen, cleaned the area and put in local anaesthetic. Then I nicked the skin and superficial muscle layers and took hold of the trocar. This is a large pointed plastic screw which penetrates the muscle layers and goes into the rumen. It is then secured into the layers by its large threads and sutured into a fixed position. The centre of this screw is removed and all the gas escapes through the remaining hollow device, much to the animal's relief. The bloated rumen applies significant pressure to the chest and also to the large veins which send blood from the hindquarters to the heart. With the gas vented, the circulation is restored to a more normal flow.

'In Germany, at this stage they say "Achtung!"' I informed Mr Morden. I had first seen this done at the Hannover Vet School. The vet at that time had positioned himself like an executioner about to wield an axe. His blow had certainly startled the beast. I was a little more restrained.

'I ken fit that means,' smiled Mr Morden. 'I just hope this beast isn't a Kraut. On you go.' And he braced himself against the calf.

I plunged the trocar in. The animal gave a little jump. Quickly I screwed the trocar in. Then I put in a couple of sutures to hold it in place. The calf began to buckle at the legs. Immediately I removed the central part of the trocar. Gas wooshed out. The calf stood up straight and took some slow deep breaths. The gas venting was methane, and highly inflammable. There were apocryphal and true stories of disasters involving folk playing with matches at this stage of the procedure.

'That looks okay to me. I will leave you with drugs to give it for at least a week. You can use the central part to clear it out if it ever gets blocked. I would check it twice a day for that. Give me a phone in a fortnight and we can discuss when is the best time to remove it.'

'Fine, fine... while you're here, Richard, I have a heifer I want you to look at. I bought it from a neighbour and I can't get it in calf. She is tied up in yon further byre for handiness. Could you have a look at her?'

'Sure,' I said. 'Usual rules,' I added, pointing to the alert collie. Mr Morden sniggered and grabbed the dog, and I nipped by with my tray of implements. Back at the car I put on my long PD gown and long plastic gloves. I marched back to the byre.

'Wait,' I said, 'let's try something.' I strode on in my long green gown. Sure enough the biting collie cowered in the corner.

'He's no fool,' volunteered Mr Morden.

'Probably not,' I agreed.

'What I meant is that he thought you were going to stick your bloody great arm up his backside,' explained Mr Morden. 'God, I've had "a doctor" do that to me and I practically jumped off the bed through the bloody wall!'

I laughed. These old boys had a direct sense of humour. We found the heifer. She seemed to be in average body condition. Mr Morden told me he had not wanted her to become too fat during her first pregnancy.

I put my hand inside her rectum and felt around. At first I could not find anything. This sometimes happens when there is a calf inside but it has dropped well forward into the depths of the abdomen. I pushed my hand in deeper: she resented this a little. Mr Morden leaned on her to stop her twirling around. Still I could find nothing. So I brought my hand all the way back and eventually found two spaghetti-thin pieces of possible womb and some minute ovaries. Then the penny dropped. I extricated my hand and looked at her rear end. The conformation of the vulva and clitoris was abnormal and a little large.

'Is she a twin?' I asked.

'Damned if I ken,' replied Mr Morden, 'but I could find out. I just bought her from a neighbour. It was a good price at the time for a breeding beast.'

'Well, I don't think she will make that,' I informed him. 'I am almost a hundred per cent certain she is a freemartin. She will never have a calf, if I am right. She would have been a twin and the other one was a male calf.'

'I ken fit you're saying,' nodded, Mr Morden. 'Damn the bit!' He spat on the floor. 'Just wait until I have a word with young Bruce.'

'I would be diplomatic… no need to rub him up the wrong way,' I said, urging caution.

'It'll be okay. It's the son, young Bruce, who sold it me. I ken the family weel. And they ken me. We'll come to some arrangement.'

'Well, if there's any doubt or if you are happy for him to speak to me, I will explain,' I added.

'Oh, there's no need for any explaining. I would put money that young lad kent fine what he was doing. He said I could either fatten or breed from her. Don't you worry, vet, it will sort.'

He said it in such emphatic tones that I left it. Sure enough I heard no more about the matter after that. As I sauntered back to the car I felt a large tug. Turning round I found the biting collie attached to the edge of my PD gown.

'Down, yer fashous brute!' shouted Mr Morden. The collie let go immediately and retreated to his usual station.

'Well, I'll be seeing you,' I said as I cleaned my boots and left.

'Nae doot,' Mr Morden replied examining his wellies. Vets did not get the 'haste ye back'.

'Vet Three to base,' I radioed in.

'Could you just go by Michie, Fieldhead, please? He has one calf he wants cut. It's more or less on your way. Neil's had to do a Caesar.'

'Okay, fine that,' I replied. The farm was just off the main road back to Inverden and was up a small slope. Why it was called "Fieldhead" after the slopes of my previous visit was a little mystery. Perhaps it was the heads of the field it referred to. Mr Michie was waiting for me. He had a bucket of warm water and a bar of soap and a towel to hand.

'It is just in here,' he said, indicating an open court with gates all around it. 'Andy has got a had of it. I'd hope you could just do this in passing,' he said, as I followed him. That was a hint that he would rather I did not charge him a full visit charge. Little did he know that it was the girls who often exercised their judgement on these matters, as they coordinated most of the visits. Those they deemed 'hassle-free' in passing probably got this reduction.

'Well, we'll see,' I said non-committally.

'There's only one because they're all supposed to have been cut. I bought this batch of stot calves last week. But this one is not cut and we think the rest are okay. But perhaps if you have time you could help us double-check the rest.'

'How many are there?' I asked the all-important question.

'Only ten,' he replied.

Without changing my expression, I was relieved. If he'd said forty I wouldn't have been too surprised. I'd brought my scalpel and artery forceps and had soon castrated the calf. The calf ran away. It is surprising how little they seem to be affected. Unlike lambs, who are given rubber rings when they are a few days old:

the ring ligates forcefully the testes and the scrotum containing them. After a short period the ligated tissue drops off harmlessly. The lambs definitely undergo a stress at the time of applying the band. One farmer pointed out that to his surprise calves, 'banded' in the same way at that same age, show little effect. This highlighted to me that there is still more research needed in these areas.

'You feel down behind them as we hold them in this wee race, vet,' advised Mr Michie. He had set up a small race and he and his two sons moved the calves through, stopping them for me to check. It all went quite smoothly. I had felt twelve scrota and no sign of any testicles. The seven others were heifer calves.

'Seems okay to me,' I told him. 'Just that other one you found at first.'

'I will need to see him about that,' Mr Michie said.

'In that case I will take the tag number of the one I just cut,' I told him. We took its number and I put it into my book in case I needed it later. I cleaned myself up and went.

'Vet Three to base,' I radioed in.

'That took you some time,' replied Emma. 'Big boy, was it? There's nothing else on.'

'In that case I will come back. He asked me to grope my way through all the other calves to check if he had any more bull calves,' I explained.

'Oh, a "while you're here",' guessed Emma.

'Something like that.'

When I arrived back at the surgery there wasn't much happening. So, it being past half past twelve, I went for lunch. At home Maya greeted me and then sped round the garden a few times while I warmed up some soup. After that I collapsed on a couch and closed my eyes: both Neil and I found a few minutes' quiet at lunchtime a very good tonic. Ten minutes later, as if on cue, the phone rang. I yawned and with my eyes still closed grabbed it.

'Yes?' I vouchsafed no politeness at this time.

'Sorry to disturb you, Richard, but a gentleman has just brought in a cat he picked up off the road. We think it's been hit by a car. Do you mind seeing it now, please?' June, in contrast, was always polite and firm.

'Right, I'll be along. Try and get all the details,' I growled.

'Of course,' responded June.

On the other end of the phone I grimaced. These sudden disturbances did no good for my stomach. Outside the fresh air woke me up. I put Maya away and headed up.

The cat was in a cat cage on a table in the consulting room. It was sitting down on its rear in a peculiar position. It appeared slightly dazed and gazed down at its chest in an introverted manner. I stood opposite and looked at it, checking its respiration rate and the style of movement of the chest. These gave good clues as to the possibility of a 'flail chest' or ruptured diaphragm. Thankfully, all appeared normal.

'Any owner?' I asked June, who was now standing beside me.

'No, but we know whereabouts it was found. The driver has gone. It looks as though it has a home. I've checked it. It doesn't appear to have a microchip.'

The phone rang in the distance. Emma came in.

'That's Mrs McClure asking after her cat. It's black and white and gone missing.'

'Oh, I think I remember this one when it came in for vaccination. It's hers, I think. Emma, ask her to come in can you?' said June.

'Well, let's see what we've got,' I remarked as I opened the top lid of the cage. The gums of the cat were not too pale. I began to listen to its torso with my stethoscope. The chest sounded fine and the intestines too. The claws were slightly shredded, a good indicator that the cat had been hit and had tried to use its claws as it landed on tarmac at speed. The back responded normally to some basic tests. I tried gently to raise the cat up on its hind legs, but it hissed and spat at me.

'I think we'll just give it a painkiller, something for shock, and an antibiotic and keep it under observation until Mrs McClure comes. Perhaps when it has steadied up a bit we can X-ray it. I suspect it has damaged hips. With a bit of luck the femurs are okay. Can you put it in a comfy cage with cat litter flat down? I don't think it can climb into a cat litter tray. We need to see if it can pee. Keep an eye on it.'

June and I attended to the injections while Emma prepared a cage.

There was no point in returning home, so I waited until the first of the afternoon appointees turned up early and saw them. After I had seen four different pet owners June waylaid me.

'Neil can finish the rest. Could you go to Strachan, Brunach? He has some beasts in a fattening court he's not very happy with. If you're not back I will get Neil to see Mrs McClure. Can you jot down on the record card what you have given it?'

'Okay... thanks, June, any idea what is worst with them?' I asked. Sometimes farmers gave clues by one or two words mentioned.

'No, he said you had better come and see them yourself.'

'Ominous,' I said.

'Be positive, Richard,' encouraged June. Vets usually had fairly fertile imaginations and have seen enough disasters to be very wary when called out to 'you had better come and see for yourself' with no extra information volunteered.

'Okay, okay. Tea on my return?'

'Of course.' June laughed.

Brunach was a neat farm; livestock was only part of the overall activities. On one side there was a large concrete apron onto which grain stores and potato stores had been built. On the other side was the section I had an interest in, a set of four large well-constructed modern farm buildings stood well set apart from each other on a small level concrete plateau. Large steel girders or beams had been sunk into the concrete in each corner and other vertical girders were spaced along each side. They reached up to a height of over fifteen metres. Walls had been made on the back by dropping railway sleepers between the vertical girders. The troughs on the front side could be mechanically filled. They also had sets of yokes by which many animals could be trapped by the head when they ate. The roof was made of some strong plastic material set at an angle with a large gap at the eaves to aid ventilation. I stopped the car on the spotlessly clean concrete. Mr Strachan came bustling towards me. He had a very business-like approach to matters and hated any problems. Whilst he was demanding, he was reasonable once a matter was clearly explained to him.

'Come with me and have a look at this,' he said.

'Is this the only building affected?' I asked.

'One is quite enough,' he replied.

We turned the corner, marching briskly toward the building. A couple of farmhands walked in a more leisurely fashion behind us.

'There.' Mr Strachan stopped, abruptly faced the building and looked at the beasts in front of him. I always wondered what some people expected of me at this stage. Even if I do suspect what the disease is I keep my councsel until I have seen a bit more. Blurting out my first thoughts handed over a few hostages to fortune. About fifty in number seven hundred-weight stirks were before me. One or two were coughing a little. About ten had weepy eyes and a clear nasal discharge. The inner corner of their eyes hinted at a slight redness, suggestive of a fever. The troughs were full of food, again suggestive of a reduced appetite.

'I can't understand how this has happened. I haven't bought anything in to this site for months,' moaned Mr Strachan.

'Have they been vaccinated?' I asked.

'Not these, they are so big I thought would be too old to get anything, and besides, I thought once they had settled down I would get away with it. You mean that IBR virus don't you?' He stuffed his hands into his pockets.

'Yes, I do. It can unfortunately strike beasts this age too. The virus is a herpesvirus. They have a tendency to go latent, hidden, and then particularly with a stress one individual can start excreting the virus and smit or infect all the others. Anything been happening here recently?'

'Yes, about a week ago someone from the Department came and insisted we check all the tags. There was a problem with the passport of one which came from the mart months ago. We had to handle them all, check every tag. It was quite a carry-on. Still, I'll get my subsidy payments, but will it help to pay for this lot of sickness? Even if none die the weight gains and feed conversions will all be down.' He pushed his hands even deeper into his pockets. 'Oh, I've got one trapped in the yokes for you at the end there,' he murmured. Mr Strachan was always very efficient.

I went up and looked at it. First I put on some latex gloves then I examined the head in some detail, this included having a good look at the eyes, the conjunctivae, the nose, and the inside of the mouth, including the tongue. Next I jumped over the yoke and checked out the rest of the body, in particular the throat, chest and related lymph glands. Finally I took its temperature: 104°F. Normal in temperate climates is from 101.5°F to 102.5°F. IBR, or Infectious Bovine Rhinotracheitis to give it its full name, seemed the most likely cause of what was happening on this site.

'Well, let's do the following, Mr Strachan. On the strength it is IBR, can you send one of your boys down to the practice for vaccine for this entire house? And I would do the other houses as well. Some may say that that is added expense: the virus doesn't often travel that distance from house to house. But with the total value of the stock here I would rather you didn't chance it. So he will need two hundred doses; Emma will give it to him. Meanwhile you, the others and I will get our hands on these affected ones and recheck it is most likely IBR. We'll treat the bad ones and take some swabs. When your boy comes back we can send him off to the lab with the swabs to confirm. I'll take blood samples from a few.'

I went back to my car and radioed Emma to tell what was brewing.

'You'll be a whiley, then?' asked Emma.

'I think I had better make sure this is done right. I'll radio when I'm finished.' Neil and I had once worked out the value of two hundred animals on a site like this; at the end of our calculation we had increased our insurance cover. A very conservative estimate would be £140,000 but then that took little account of subsidies and other matters which meant it could be twice as much.

I returned to the yard. Mr Strachan had given up on getting the beasts trapped in the yokes. He and other staff had placed a crush in the building and set up sets of gates. We put the worst-looking animals in first. They all had temperatures and signs consistent with IBR. A cough, and a clear or pussy nasal and eye discharge could be observed in some of them. One or two had small erosions in their nose or on the palate. I beavered away, examining the stirks, noting down tag numbers and taking blood samples and swabs from four, treating them with long-acting antibiotics, vitamin E and selenium, and an anti-inflammatory. It was at the early stage of the outbreak, so after about eight I stopped and waited for the vaccine. The remaining mild or very early cases can often be treated with the IBR vaccine alone. This live vaccine has the remarkable side effect of stimulating the rapid production of interferon. This helps greatly in damping down the severity of these virus disease outbreaks.

The vaccine arrived. I also injected with an antibiotic any odd individual I was not too happy with. The vaccine is made up of ten millilitres of solution in a vial. The syringe is loaded with two millilitres and then the needle is taken off. In its place a one and a half-inch plastic nozzle is positioned. One person secures the head while another person inserts the nozzle up the nose and shoots the two mililitres high up into the nose. It is not painful, but the stirks tend to wriggle a bit.

Once we had finished that house I looked at the other cattle. They showed no signs of illness. Then I instructed them to disinfect their clothes before they vaccinated the other houses. It was probably best to do it first thing tomorrow, I suggested. I might well have a lab result by then. They were not too sure how to disinfect themselves so we all trooped off to the power hose.

'This is how you do it,' I said. I started to spray myself and splash on disinfectant. Eyebrows were raised at the thoroughness. But then they soon joined in and soaked each other.

'So long as you're clean it doesn't matter,' I said.

'I think you had better bugger off before we sort you out too,' one of them said with a laugh.

'You okay, Mr Strachan?' I asked.

'Aye, aye you can bugger off, as he said. Thanks a lot for your time. I'll vaccinate next year.'

'I'll drop round tomorrow, I'll phone to arrange a suitable time for both of us.'

'Fine that, see you.' His head was down, concentrating on cleaning himself.

'Bye!' I drove off, my car receiving a gargantuan douche.

'Vet Three to base.'

'Ah, Richard, Mr Michie wondered if you are passing if you could drop by. The calf you cut this morning is bleeding a bit. I think you had better check it,' said Emma.

'Righto,' I replied. In twenty minutes I was back at Michie's.

'Thanks for coming. Perhaps it's not as bad as I thought.' He gave me a weak smile.

'Better be safe,' I said. 'Mind you, this doesn't often happen on young calves such as this. It will be interesting to see.'

We went indoors and found the calf. There was some blood across its hindquarters, but nothing too bad. We stopped and watched it. There was no dripping of blood. We went round the pens looking for blood on the ground. All we found was one large clot.

'I think it's best to leave it,' I advised. 'There may have been a gathering in the bag and when that was released it gave the impression of significant bleeding. I agree, much better to check these things. But with no blood coming out at the moment we had best leave it. If I tinker with it now it could cause infection or make it worse.'

'Fine, fine. Well, you're the professional,' said Mr Michie. 'I forgot to mention it this morning. Could you look at my collie bitch? She has lumps down below. She's a fair age. Bess, come by!' he hollered. A fit but very unkempt collie turned up. He held her head while I felt around her belly. At first I encountered clods of dried dirt and mud welded into her hair. But Mr Michie said he knew about those. Feeling deeper, I found the body of the dog and sure enough there were growths in her mammary glands on the left side.

'Aye, you're right,' I concurred. 'It would be better to remove those growths. If she's up to it, we can strip off all the mammary glands on one side. That will sort it, I hope. At any rate, it'll give her a fighting chance. Can you shear her belly first, before the surgeon gets his hands on her? Anne is a bit fussy and doesn't like to do a grooming before the op.'

'What a cheek!' Mr Michie laughed. Farmers could usually take a bit of a dig at them. 'Do I stop feeding her before the operation?'

'Aye. The night before – no food. Phone Emma or June to arrange to do this in the next fortnight. They'll fill you with the latest details. Oh, and she won't be working for at least four weeks after the op. I am not having her flying over a barbed-wire fence two days after the op with stitches on her belly.' I wanted to give the bitch some recuperation.

'Okay, fine,' said Mr Michie, and ruffled the hair of his collie with genuine concern. I nipped into my car and away.

'Vet Three to base.'

'Nothing else,' replied June.

'Righto. I'm coming back.'

I shoved a CD in and found an apple to chew on. Once I was back at the surgery there was a lot of tidying up to do. Syringes and needles had to be disposed of, drugs to be replenished, and worst of all a pile of administration to work through. It went on and on. Although pharmacists do not record in detail batch numbers of the medicines that they give to humans, vets have to note these numbers down for all the farm animals they treat. Neil was in a corner cursing a ministry form linked to samples taken from a cow that aborted. He had to note a date down in no less than four places on one piece of paper. When he had finished that he had to send another official form to the farmer instructing him to isolate the cow. The irony of all this is that while in the last ten years the paperwork for these abortion investigations has increased, the practical work has gone down in standard. Before as a standard the swab sample from the aborted cow was checked for brucella and salmonella. Now it is only checked for brucella. Both diseases are zoonoses: diseases which can cause serious disease in man.

Soon the small animal clients were coming in. Neil, Anne and I shared the load. With three vets and two consulting rooms we could work efficiently.

'Mrs Baillie for you, Richard,' June said. Emma had by now left to leave June to finish the day.

Mrs Baillie and I entered the consulting room. Outside it was completely dark. One or two raindrops ran down the window. The room was a little haven compared to the wild weather outside.

'He's not keen on going out on nights like this, so it was easy for me to catch him tonight. It's his ears. He's been bothered with them before but that was a long time ago. I have also run out of drops,' she informed me as she dropped the cage on the table. A muted mew came from inside objecting, no doubt, to the style of handling. I noted that his record showed he had been treated twice before. 'Jasper is his name,' she added.

I removed the black cat from the cage. He scanned the whole room in a furtive manner with his head and neck crouched low. I pulled up an ear flap and saw that dark debris filled the outer ear. All the signs suggested ear mites. Using a cotton bud I extracted some of the mess and shook a bit onto a microscope slide. Muttering an excuse, I went next door and put the slide on the platform of the microscope. Sure enough, there were mites present. I centred one in the middle of the field of vision and invited Mrs Baillie in for a viewing. She gasped with amazement at the sight of the eight-legged creature waddling across the field of view. He was climbing over dark boulders of microscopic debris. The mite was disc-shaped with a few individual long hairs sticking out near his odd, conically shaped legs. He seemed to be making a great deal of effort for the little distance he was travelling. Then, as so many owners had done before, Mrs Baillie turned away from the microscope and looked at Jasper. She was finding it hard to believe that at that very moment living inside the two small ears of the cat there were a great number of minute creatures.

'It's incredible to think he's full of those beasties!' she said.

I took some eardrops off the shelf and treated Jasper. Then I quickly closed the cage door before he shook his head vigorously and dispersed a fine spray of mites, eardrop solution and debris around the area. Mrs Baillie exited, holding the cat cage like a trophy and smiling.

I took three more cases and then we had all finished. I saw Anne take up the practice mobile phone. She was on duty that night. One of the hardest things after completing a day's work is to be faced with a night on duty. It can on occasion be like starting a whole day's work again. I said my goodbyes and headed for home. I was looking forward to a glass of sherry.

Chapter Eight

The longest night.

The next morning I went into the surgery to find a large number of surgical instruments laid across a surface in one of the prep rooms. Anne was obviously tidying up after operating on a cow. It looked like a Caesar kit. She appeared slightly ruffled.

'My seven a.m. wake up call,' she explained. 'Mind you, I don't mind that so much. It's the three o'clock to five o'clock ones that I don't like at all. Then I'm not fit for anything the next day.' I kept silent.

That day progressed much as the day before. One or two matters spilled over from yesterday. I checked Mr Strachan's stirks. They were all back eating, so we left them alone and by the time I had arrived the stockmen had vaccinated all the other stirks. The lab report had come back. It was positive for IBR. The fluorescent antibody tests were very quick in producing a result. The result had been waiting in the fax machine when I went in to work. Mr Michie had phoned to say the calf was fine but he would like a short statement typed out by me concerning the calf, the fact that it had been entire and that I had castrated it.

Evening came and it was my turn on duty. I diverted the telephone through to my house and then using another phone dialled the practice number.

'Hello?' It was Jill.

'You've got the phones – I'm coming down now, okay?' I said.

'Yes, fine,' she replied.

By the time I'd arrived someone had phoned.

'Jimmy Geddes phoned. He has got a heifer with a prolapse. He's just calved her,' announced Jill as I came in. I looked at the table with the supper on it. 'You could take a bite now. I'm sure one minute won't make a difference.'

'No, I'd better go,' I said. 'Besides, it may be quite hard work and I might bring that up.' I nodded at the lasagne. Edward turned up his nose

'Oh, Dad, you're terrible!' But I had gone.

Jimmy was about six miles down the main road. His farm was beyond some woods off the road. I drove round past a large silo to some pens at the back. There I found he had put the heifer up a race and into a crush out in the open. Fortunately it was not raining and the heifer was alert and standing. An enormous pink protuberance hung from her rear. It was her uterus – but everted out from the abdomen. On rare occasions after the appearance of the calf the dam continues to press and strain. The result is that sometimes the womb comes out as well. If it's not replaced soon, the mother will die.

'It is only just out, and not too big,' Jimmy encouraged me.

I put on my PD gown and faced behind the heifer. First I cleared excess placenta off the womb. Then I sprinkled the womb with sugar, which by osmosis often shrinks it. Another farmhand came beside me, and using three fists we began to push this enormous pink and red object back into a small hole. This required a large amount of effort. The PD gown does not 'breathe' so I became very hot. Bit by bit, more and more of the womb slowly disappeared into the heifer. She, however, began to press to try and foil our hard work. By careful coordination of our fists we always made sure that there was one fist in the vagina acting as a valve to stop any womb reappearing outside again. Finally we got it all in. Time goes slowly on these occasions, so that although it seemed an age it had in fact only been about four minutes' hard work. I asked for a bottle and using it as a blunt extension of my arm I ensured that the womb was well back and in place. Then I placed an enormous tight suture at the back to stop a recurrence, gave her some antibiotics, calcium and vitamins, and left her. Jimmy opened the front of the crush, she exited and looked around for her calf.

Near my car was a trough and a tap. Using these I cleaned the worst of the blood and faeces off my gown and kit.

'I think she'll be okay,' I told Jimmy. 'We got it back quickly. There has been little damage, if any, to the womb, and she doesn't appear to be shocked at all.'

'Fine,' he replied. He was a man of few words. I left and after a mile or so stopped and used the phone.

'Anything doing?' I asked Jill.

'No.'

'Well, I'll just go back to the surgery to use the hose and get some buckets of warm water to really clean up. Then I'll be home.'

Twenty minutes later I was back home and eating a warmed-up supper. The children had disappeared up to the computer room, never to be seen again that evening. I read a newspaper, watched a programme on TV and then began to head for bed. The first action, paradoxically, was to put the dog out for a few minutes. Just then the phone rang. Jill came through with the phone.

'It's a Graeme. I can't catch the name of the farm,' she passed it to me.

'Hello?' I said non-committally.

'That you, Richard?' said Graeme, and before I could reply he carried on. ' I am at the steading on the hill – you know, up by Merchlan.'

'I know,' I said with little enthusiasm.

'Well, I've got a cow at the calving and she's not getting down to it at all. The feet seem very big. I think I would be better with the help of a vet.'

'Righto,' I said, 'I'll come now. Can you make sure there are two buckets of clean warm water ready when I arrive? That's in case it's a Caesar.'

'Sure, I'll go down to Jean's now and have it ready by the time you get here,' he said.

I put the phone down. The steading was halfway up Ben Aich on a deserted hill farm. Graeme, who was of pensionable age, went up there to check the cows every night. I could just imagine the steading enshrouded in mist high up that hill. The nearest human habitation was a mile and a half down the brae. Jean, a vet who had helped out with our small animal work from time to time, lived there with her husband, Edward. I told Jill I was off and would almost certainly be quite some time. It was eleven miles to the foot of the hill from our house.

I arrived at the turn off from the main road and started the climb up the hill, following a thin single-file metalled road. After a quarter of a mile I passed two occupied farmhouses and a turning to another farm. Then I was all alone. The road continued to rise and crossed a cattle grid with a small plantation of conifers away to my left. Just before the cattle grid a small road end could be seen. It was the end of Jean's farm track. The road now hugged the side of the hill, wending its way in and out of gullies like a sheep track. On one side I had the grass of the hill's slope while on the other a significant drop. The road was wet so I drove with caution.

Soon the visibility reduced to twenty yards with the result that I came upon another cattle grid by surprise, hearing it before I saw it. I knew this to be the last one before the farm buildings, which would be at the end of a straight section of road. These buildings I knew to be in the dip between two large hilltops. From this site, which amounted to the mid point of a ridge, you could see into the valleys on either side of the hills. But tonight, all I could see was the faint light coming from over the closed part of a half-heck door of the buildings. This door was in the corner of the building that was shaped like an 'L'. A concrete platform about three feet high led up to the door. This platform was used to load animals out from the byre directly onto a cattle truck. On one side of the platform was the building while on the other were a set of posts with fence rails. They had all seen better days. As I walked across the platform to the light I could see green algae present at the base of the posts and growing across the concrete. The posts, which were a little rotten, were covered in algae and lichen; the average humidity here was high. A gutter hanging down from its moorings drained rain out from its unsecured end. It only served to confirm the dilapidated state of this farm building.

I leant my torso over the open part of the half-heck door into the building. Three naked light bulbs illuminated the large room, which was about eighteen by eight yards wide. In contrast to the outside this room was dry, relatively warm, and light. It was good to see human beings there: three. It may appear trite, but in a circumstance such as this company makes the difficulties bearable. Graeme, his wife Pat and Jean looked at me expectantly. I paused for a second and smiled. It was good to see them. I could see from their look that we had a problem, and so decided to mimic Duncan's brevity.

'Hi,' I said.

'*Hello*,' they replied in chorus. I paused one more second and then cut through the air of drama.

'Well, we had better just see what we've got.' I knew Graeme well enough to know that he would not call me out for some minor matter.

'I think the calf is on the wee bitty large side. But ye'll ken; you're the expert.'

The last phrase was one I dreaded. Experts can be wrong, as the media are always willing to point out.

'I've got her round in the next room, the byre with four stalls. She is tied up for handiness and I've given her a bottle of calcium under the skin.'

I followed Graeme to the next room, a very cosy wee byre with four stalls. The large black cow looked at me nervously. I had my PD gown on and put my hand inside to assess the situation. Right enough, the calf was large. However, the front feet and the head were all in the right place. She was a big cow.

'You haven't given her a pull or anything like that?' I asked.

'No, I just left her to it. The waters were off sometime after lunch. I took her in about six and gave her some calcium. Perhaps I should have done something then but I didn't want to upset her. She hadn't been pressing and I hoped that she would calve. She wasn't fully, fully open then.'

'Aye. It's difficult to say, isn't it? Well, we have got to do something now, so I suggest we try with the machine. I like to give them a chance rather than Caesar everything. But if it's too stiff we'll just have to resort to the knife, sad to say.'

'Aye… aye, it's surprising what they can produce when they really push. Shall we move her next door for using the machine? It's bit tight for her here. What if she goes down?' Graeme asked.

'Aye, fine, that. I will just get my machine and the ropes.'

I returned to my car and extracted the calving aid. It's a crank mechanism which can with some force pull a calf out from the cow. Graeme and the others had meanwhile placed a halter on the cow and moved her into the room away from the byre. The cow was tied by a rope to a secure lug on the wall. I put my hand inside her to position the ropes on the calf's front feet just above the fetlocks. The cow skipped a bit, so both she and I danced a little across the floor; then she settled down. Next we all took up our positions. We had all done this enough times to know our roles. I kept my hand inside the pelvis to ascertain what progress the calf was making in coming out. Graeme worked the ratchet handle of the calving aid under my instruction. Jean held the base of the calving aid hard into a position just below the pelvic brim of the cow. On occasion the base of the machine could slip sideways or down. It was vital to halt this type of movement. Pat kept her hand on the far end of the calving aid to make sure it was angled correctly and therefore pulling in the right direction.

'Okay start it up,' I told Graeme.

He began to take in a few strokes of the ratchet. The calf moved a bit. We waited. The cow pressed a little. Graeme ratcheted a bit more. The calf moved a little. The cow strained a lot and bellowed. The calf hardly moved. Graeme tried a little more 'pressure'. A little more movement came. The head was in the correct position but it felt very tight. There was a minute amount of room for my hand. With my spare hand I felt the tension on the ropes. They were very taut. In the back of my mind alarm bells were beginning to ring.

'Well, just see if she can push it a little more,' I said. The cow heaved a great push but the calving ropes still remained very taut. I knew we could theoretically pull the calf out, but there was a significant risk of damage to both cow and calf. Although I was halfway up a hill in Scotland, I reckoned I had to choose another option.

'Right,' I said. 'I'm sorry, but I've had enough of that. It's all too tight. We would very likely kill the calf,even damage her. We'll just have to do a Caesar,'

'I thought so,' said Graeme. Like me, he was disappointed that we could not calve her. But also like me, he knew we had little choice.

This is the point when every veterinary surgeon has to demonstrate mental strength and flexibility. For the previous twenty minutes he or she has been attempting the veterinary equivalent of a pole vault. He has been using a machine to produce a coordinated movement: the delivery of the calf using the correct application of strength, timing, positioning, balance. This movement has also to be completed allowing for the fact that the helpers may or may not understand your instructions, and the cow may move suddenly in a variety of directions. All at once this 'pole vault' is abandoned in a volte-face, and the vet has a completely different mission.

Firstly he or she must now create an operating theatre in or around the location. This in my case was a byre halfway up a Scottish hill. Secondly he or she must carry out a piece of surgery with speed and dexterity. This is the largest mammalian surgical operation that is carried out on a daily basis throughout Britain. The mother weighs seven or more times the weight of an average human being, and the offspring is ten to fifteen times the weight of a human baby.

I packed away my calving equipment and fished two well-laden large plastic trays from my car. All my kit for a Caesarean section was in them. On reentering the room I found Graeme and Pat spreading out fresh straw to make a semblance of basic hygiene. Jean and I went to a corner and laid out all the pieces. The first tray had all the preparation material. The second held all the instruments and drugs for the operation. Once we had them all ready, I turned to face the cow holding two loaded syringes. I had a headlamp on. Graeme pinched the cow's nose to steady her and I injected two drugs into her jugular vein. One would make her almost comatose but not fully anaesthetised. The other would affect the tone of the uterus to make surgery less tricky.

We watched her and sure enough our luck was in. She began to buckle at the feet, straightened herself up a couple of times and then collapsed in a heap, snoring deeply.

With minimal exchanges we all set to work. Graeme and Pat tied the front feet together and then tied them to a gatepost, extending the legs slightly. They then tied the hocks together tightly and pulled the hind legs back to another secure post. Next they tied the head down to make sure she could not raise it. One of them then sat on the upper part of the neck away from the windpipe to ensure she didn't move at a critical point. Meanwhile Jean and I had injected the left side of the abdomen with local anaesthetic. Then we cleaned the area thoroughly using one of the buckets of clean water laced with disinfectant. Next we applied an iodine and alcohol mix followed by a large drape. We were almost ready to start. Jean and I scrubbed up with the other bucket.

'All ready?' I asked. They nodded. 'Well, here goes, she may flinch a bit to start with, but once we are through the skin she'll probably settle down.'

I cut a hole in the drape to reveal the skin. Then I checked my landmarks on the cow and made an incision in the skin. The cow moved, but as I had predicted, settled down as I quickly went through more muscle layers. A flow of blood came from these layers; I ignored these unless they were copious. By the end of the operation they would have stopped. Time was of the essence. We had to keep moving for our goal. I came across the exterior of the peritoneum. It was a thin membrane holding in the abdominal contents. With care I nicked it and exposed a small opening into the cavern of the abdomen. Using a finger I carefully enlarged the hole with a pair of scissors.

'We're in,' I said. 'Now, let's see if we can find the womb. Jean, can you arm yourself with a scalpel, please?'

The nice fact of having Jean around was that she was a surgeon too, albeit with smaller animals and used to far more delicate tissues than the ones I regularly handled. She stood beside me holding the scalpel like an item of some religious significance. I found the womb and felt around it until I could detect a foot inside. Then with a heave I guided it towards the opening we had created. The force required to do this is large, and I had to be careful not to put my fingers through the womb. It is usually impossible to raise the piece of womb very high. In this case I got it to just level with the opening.

'Now, Jean, make a bold incision between my hands. It will be over the hoof,' I instructed.

Jean did this well; many farmers are a little wary of helping in that cut. Quickly, I pushed my hand through the hole she had created, found a hoof and pulled it through the small hole. Jean had a rope to hand and we tied it on. Then we opened the womb incision a little more and I found the other foot, which we also secured with a rope. The incision in the womb was still not large enough for the calf to come out, so I ordered Graeme and Jean to begin to pull the calf out slowly, while with blunt pointed scissors I enlarged the womb incision to a size just large enough for the calf. We then used a large amount of force to lift the calf up as vertically as possible out of the cow. It came quite easily, and we put him down on the cow's side with the cord intact. Quickly I started to get him to breathe, injecting him with two respiratory stimulants and poking a piece of straw up his nose to stimulate him to sneeze. He sneezed, blinked, and the sides of his chest started to go up and down.

At a certain point we decided to cut him from his mother. So we clamped his navel and pulled him to one side and put him in a corner. Graeme kept an eye on him while Jean and I returned to the cow. The hard work had just begun. We now had to tidy the cow up and sew back pieces we had cut. I pulled out as much placenta as possible. Infected placental contents in a cow five days post operation are potentially lethal. Then we placed some pessaries of antibiotics in the womb. Jean had threaded a large needle and catgut for me. We sewed the womb up carefully. It's a tricky job, since it's slippery and able to change shape all the time. It was important to make sure that the wound line, once sewn up, had a good 'seal'. Once that was completed I returned the womb to its rightful position and double-checked that it was snugly in the correct part of the abdomen. We placed a little more antibiotic in the part of the abdomen where we had been active. Then we began to sew up the three muscle layers and the peritoneum. This always appears to take an age, however quick one goes, and even if one sews two layers together. Finally we came to the skin. I used a set of needle holders to grip the cutting needle with vigour. The needle has to go through hide, which in the living animal is tough and flexible. This was completed without event. I looked behind; the calf was blinking and offering to rise up.

Jean started tidying up while I went round and did all my post-op checks. I checked the birth canal of the cow; I needed to be sure that the placenta could be passed with ease. Sometimes I found a piece of placenta inside which I then guided and pulled into the birth canal. I gave the cow some oxytocin to hasten the involution of the womb. Finally she received an antibiotic injection and another bottle of calcium. Next I went to the calf to check his navel, which I dipped in iodine. I also gave him an antibiotic injection, since a very high percentage of Caesar claves get neonatal infections.

Graeme assured me he would guarantee that the calf received the colostrum. This is the first milk, full of antibodies; without receiving this milk in the first twelve to twenty-four hours of life, the calf would probably die as it would have a seriously compromised immune system. We propped the cow up so that she could belch. If she was unable to belch her rumen could blow up to such an extent that she too would die. She looked a little groggy, but considering what she had undergone I thought she was fine. I thought that Graeme would start to milk colostrum from her but instead he turned to me.

'That's good, Richard. But I wonder if you could look at something for me...' Without Pat seeing, I looked at Jean and raised my eyebrows. As vets, we knew that anything could be coming next.

'I've got this cow in here—' he pointed to a small door that I had been unaware of— 'I thought she was going to calve tonight too. Well, it's night now, but she has not pressed or anything. Her water bags have not burst but her udder is full of milk. The only odd thing she does is kick a little... and look at her side.' I had a sinking feeling.

'Perhaps it's the calf inside her kicking around and upsetting her,' volunteered Pat. She was hinting that nothing was ado. Jean said nothing. I had learnt enough to be worried. This story I had heard before. Still, I was not going to mention my suspicion to any of them. Maybe it was some little glitch and all we had to do was let her get on with it.

'I think I had better check her too, seeing as I'm here. I wouldn't want you to phone me in a couple of hours' time,' I said trying to make a joke of it.

'Right, right,' said Graeme. He opened the small door. It was just a black hole. Somewhere in there was a cow.

'I'll go in,' volunteered Graeme. 'She kens me.' He disappeared into the void. Soon a cow came out. She took a couple of quick paces out, stopped, and blinked in the unaccustomed glare of three naked light bulbs. Graeme followed and sidled around her. She looked anxiously at the reception committee.

'Graeme, can you get a halter on her?' I asked in genuine concern.

'I should be able to manage,' he said, and turned for a halter. Then he approached her, speaking softly. We all stood well back. He knew her and so she stood immobile while he positioned the halter. Then he secured her to a lug on the wall. I approached her and placed my hand into the birth canal. My worst fears were confirmed.

'Damn,' I said, 'I don't believe it!'

'What?' they all looked at me as though we were in a Brian Rix farce.

'She has a twisted womb. There's probably not enough room in this building to roll her, and we can't roll her outside. Even then rolling her won't always succeed. I don't want to roll her and cause all that stress and then have to Caesar her. It's tricky; we'll be wise after the event.' In the middle of the night my trains of thought, while logical, were not easy to communicate.

'So if the womb is twisted the calf cannot get out, is that it?' asked Graeme.

'Yes,' said Jean, 'that's about it. It's not too common in cattle and almost unheard of in cats and dogs. Unfortunately, it's a high-risk situation.' She looked at me. I could see that she understood we had a problem.

'So what do we do?' asked Graeme.

'Well,' I sighed, 'I think we should just get on and Caesar her. We may be lucky and it may be fairly fresh inside. That is important, as if it has gone on for a long time the womb is impossible to sew up again. It just falls apart in your hand because it's too soft.'

'Right, well, I'll go with you, vet,' said Graeme. 'If it's a Caesar then, that is the best we can do now. We just do it.'

'Right, fine. We're all agreed. Now how do we do this?' I looked at them and round to the animals in the room. 'Okay, Jean, do you mind, can you go back down to your house and boil and resterilise my instruments? While you are doing that, Graeme, Pat and I will move the calf and the first cow next door. Oh, can you also bring up a supply of clean fresh water, please?'

'Yes, sure, I'll get on with that. I will get Ted out too. I think we need some fresh legs.'

Ted was Jean's husband. She disappeared and we heard her drive away. We then started moving the calf next door into the byre. Graeme made a little pen with plenty of straw, gated off. This was to stop the mother falling on the calf. He and I picked the calf up and gently settled him down. The cow could not move by herself so we made a carpet of straw and slid her over the ground into the byre. We propped her up and left her in a contented position. I took another tray from my car and prepared my syringes and disinfectants for the next operation. We had a minute or two to catch our breath before Jean returned.

'Here, I brought some coffee and a husband. In that order of usefulness!' She was carrying a thermos and some mugs. Ted came behind. He was a big quiet man and very practical. We all had a quick cup and then set to.

Once again I injected the cow with a heavy sedative. Down she went. While Jean and I finalised our instruments, Pat and Graeme tied the cow down. Ted gave help where required. We cleaned the side of the beast and applied drapes.

'Here we go again,' I said. I cut down through the skin and the muscle layers. Jean was standing beside me. When I cut through the final layer a gush of clear serous fluid ran down the flank of the cow.

'Don't worry, that's to be expected,' I informed them. 'In these cases many of the body fluids are in some imbalance. So we get fluids here and sometimes oedema in the wall of the womb. We'll just have to see how it goes.'

I felt around the womb. Moving my hand back to the rear I could feel the twist of the womb just around the cervix. I tried to lift the womb up but it was immobile. Furthermore, I thought it might be damaged by more handling. Once it was empty of a calf it would twist back easily to its correct position.

'Problems?' asked Jean.

'A little. I'll have to poke my hand through the womb in a case like this. I will do it just opposite a hoof and then we'll raise the hoof and try to complete the cut on the womb,' I explained.

They all watched. There was in fact nothing for them to see. My hand was deep inside the abdomen of the cow. I found a hoof. I hated to do my next action. Firstly it was a little crude and secondly there was a slight risk of losing the hole I had made inside the vast territory of the abdomen. Some surgeons would take a guarded knife in to the abdomen in these circumstances. I had tried it once and found it too hair-raising. Instead I managed to poke a finger through the wall of the uterus and then with my hand I expanded the break a little. I grasped a hoof. It was covered in foetal membranes and was slippery. The calf kicked and I lost my grip. I swore and sweat broke out on my brow immediately. Quickly I searched around and found the hoof again. This time with another hand I broke down the membranes surrounding the hoof. They seemed amazingly tough. Then, using all my strength, I pulled the hoof up, making sure I didn't lose my grip. Jean was right beside me with a rope to hand to put around the fetlock. As soon as she saw the foot she deftly secured it.

'Jean, just put a little pressure on that and I will open the womb a bit with these scissors.'

'Fine, I've got it,' she said.

I opened the womb carefully. Now it was almost outside the abdomen I could have a better view of my site of operation. I made sure that no other abdominal organ was in the way of the cut.

'Right, Jean, you can slacken a little. I'll find the other hoof by following my hand down the leg we have got.' Jean slackened a little. The foot and womb descended into the abyss. I felt down and soon found the other leg. Once it was up, Jean soon had a rope on it.

'Okay, I think we're ready to go. Ted, can you give Jean a hand with the ropes?' They pulled. This time the calf came straight out. We didn't bother with the navel cord, which broke immediately. The calf was alive and blinking but had difficulty breathing. In this condition, with all the fluid imbalances, they often have a lot of fluid on the lungs. We lifted him up to a gate and hung him by his hindquarters from the bars. Fluid came running down out of his nose.

'Come on, calfy!' urged Graeme. I was busy injecting the calf with respiratory stimulants. Jean was poking a piece of straw up his nose while Ted was rubbing his chest with vigour. The calf coughed a little. I put my hand inside his mouth and cleared the airways. I knew there were revival kits for inflating chests but we did not use them. Keeping these kits clean and using them correctly was a problem. Instead, I used a lamb catheter tube if I was completely stuck.

'Stop, let's see what he can do,' I ordered. We all went still while the calf craned his neck up and his sides started to go in and out as breathing started in earnest.

'It's a bull calf – which is good news for someone,' observed Graeme.

'I think he'll be all right. Just keep him hung up there for another couple of minutes, Ted. Rub him occasionally. Any problems give us a shout. Jean and I had better get back to the mother.'

We both went to a bucket to clean our hands then went back to the comatose cow. One or two shreds of afterbirth hung out of the abdominal incision. I used these to guide me back to the womb. I felt around for the twist. I manipulated the womb and untwisted it. Next I found my incision on the womb and brought it up to the surface of the abdomen. Then Jean and I managed to position it on the edge so we could sew it back together. It all looked fine.

'Well, this is the moment of truth,' I announced. 'Is the wall of the womb soft or no?' I tried a couple of passes through the womb and pulled them tight. Thankfully they held. The suture material did not cheese-wire through the uterus wall.

'Oh, I think we're in business here,' I declared. Jean and I rapidly sewed up the cow and put all the medicines and stitches back in their correct places. The calf bawled. I smiled; this had definitely been worth it.

Ted let it down and checked its navel. He found an apron of straw for it to lie on, and Jean told him what medicines to give it. We finished this cow faster than the first. No doubt we all wanted our beds. I performed all my checks, gave a bottle of calcium, some pituitrin, and some antibiotic to the cow. Then I also checked that the placenta could be passed. I noticed how the birth canal now was completely normal. There was no hint of the twist that had been there before. We began to tidy up. Graeme promised that he'd be up tomorrow to ensure the calves got a good amount of colostrum before lunchtime. We made a pen for the calf to protect it from the cow when she rose. After coming round from the sedative she could still be so unsteady that she might by accident fall on the calf.

'Well, I can only thank you all,' I said, 'for help in tricky circumstances. I'm off – see you.'

'Bye!' they all said.

I led the cars down off the hill. In my wing mirror I saw Jean and Ted turn off into their farm track. Clouds of mist now blew up the mountain slowing my descent; rabbits scuttled away from the headlights.

Soon I was racing back home. I had just entered the last straight stretch of road before Inverden when the mobile phone beside me rang. I braked hard and grabbed the phone.

'Yes, it's me?' I answered.

'Richard, where have you been? I haven't had a wink of sleep!' Jill asked.

'I'm sorry, but I had to do two Caesars there. I thought it was too late to phone and tell you what was happening. It's past two now.'

'Yes, well, I'm sorry but David Duthey phoned just now. He has a heifer calving. One of his pedigrees. He thinks it's almost a certain Caesar.'

'Well, I'm just opposite his road end,' I replied. By now I was past any pain barrier. 'I guess you'll see me when you see me.'

'Yes, good luck.'

'Thanks.' I reversed the car twenty yards to David's road end, turned the car up the track and soon was at the farm building. I went in. David's wife, Mary, was standing with a towel in hand and two buckets of clean hot water beside her. Just behind her stood Dod, the long-serving stockman. Even at this time of night they appeared relaxed. Of David there was no sign.

'Hello,' I said.

'Oh hello, Richard. Ah, here's David.'

David came in. He looked taken aback.

'Goodness, you're quick! I'm only just off the phone.' He was genuinely surprised.

'My wife phoned me when I was almost opposite your road end, so I stopped.'

'Ah, that's it, then,' said David. 'I saw a car on the straight suddenly slam on its brakes as I put the phone down. I get a good view from the window. I wondered what someone was doing racing down there at that time of night! But it was you heading for home.'

'Too right,' I laughed. 'Anyway, what have you got for me?'

'Oh, it's a certain Caesar. I've had a bit of a go myself. You can have a go if you want, but I doubt very much you'll succeed.' David's judgement was usually excellent. I had only ever calved one which he wanted a Caesar for, and that had been luck.

'Tell you what, I've just come from a Caesar or two.' At that time of night my tongue had loosened a little to boast. 'Mary, could you boil up my instruments? I have them in a tray. Just boil them for five minutes in a large saucepan and then drain off the water. While you're doing that I'll check this heifer and most likely prepare for an op.'

'Fine.' David smiled.

I went to my car and handed the tray over to Mary. Then I went into David's calving pen. It was a very professional affair. An area about eight metres by eight with one gate for moving cows round and a whole series of holds set into the walls for ropes. The lighting was excellent. The concrete was clean. There was clean straw all over. The heifer had already been roped down on her side with her left flank up. She was trussed up ready for the operation; David was very organised and efficient. I put my hand inside her. It all felt very tight. I wasn't going to risk one of David's good pedigree calves now. Better to play safe.

'Righto. Farmer is usually right. We're doing a Caesar. I'll just get my other bits and pieces.'

There were already two buckets of clean water standing to attention by the wall. I returned with my kit, sedated the heifer and began to prepare the flank with local anaesthetic and disinfectant. The drape went on and soon I was ready. All I needed was the instruments. David had scrubbed himself up. He was a very handy assistant.

Mary came racing down. She presented me with the instruments in the saucepan. I found a new scalpel blade and placed it onto the handle. It was very hot.

'Oh, Mary, you're hot tonight!' I joked. I was a little dizzy

'Now, young Jones,' smiled David, 'you just concentrate on the job in hand and leave my wife out of this.' I took the hint, stood up, took a deep breath, and bent down to start.

For the third time that night I cut through the skin. The heifer was smaller than the previous two. It was thus a much quicker operation. Soon we were in the abdomen. David was standing beside me with a scalpel blade and scissors to hand. One other factor that helped in this operation was having a farmer who had confidence in the vet and who gave the vet a reasonable operating area. As it was a smaller animal I was able to manipulate the womb more easily. I found the hock of the calf and grabbed that and a fetlock. Then I manoeuvred the whole conceptus up to the abdominal incision. Soon I had a piece of intact womb sticking out of the wound. There was a calf hoof below the intact uterine wall. I wished all Caesars were as easy as this to manipulate… David passed me the blade. I cut down and made one complete and sufficient opening in the womb. David and I quickly put down the scissors and the knife. We soon had ropes on the calf's fetlocks. We were able to give a very measured and quick pull. Soon we had the calf resting on the flank of the heifer. The cord was intact. Mary, who is very good at resuscitation, injected the calf with the respiratory stimulants. Dod pushed a piece of straw up its nose. The calf woke up immediately. It shook its head, flicked its floppy ears about, blinked and started breathing with vigour.

'That's okay,' said David.

I cut the navel cord and clamped it. Mary and Dod took it over to their calf area. David and I cleaned ourselves up again. Then we went into the abdomen, found the womb and returned it to the surface. I took out as much placenta as possible and placed some pessaries in the interior of the womb. Then David held the womb while I sewed it up. Mary occasionally gave advice on my stitching. Some vets would take exception to this, but I knew Mary to be a sewing expert. Besides, I knew them well enough to know there was no malice intended. In a surprisingly short time, the job was done. All the usual checks were made. At the same time as we had been sewing up the heifer, Dod had milked her and had placed a good amount of colostrum in a jug. He and David then moved to the calf, stomach-tubed it and poured all the colostrum into its stomach. He injected the calf and treated its navel. Just as we finished the heifer got up. On occasion, some do get up quick.

'Well, that's fine,' said David. 'I think you'd better go to bed.'

'That is not a bad idea. I'll see you – bye,' I said, and I headed off.

'You were quick!' whispered Jill. 'Did you calve it, then?'

'No, I Caesared it,' I replied.

'Speedy.'

No, not really,' I demurred. 'David had everything set up perfectly. Still, I was nowhere near Stuart Imray's record forty-five minutes on and off.'

'Well, whatever. You had better try and get some sleep.'

'Right.' I just dozed off.

Next morning I got up and felt rough. It was going to be a difficult day. Usually after a long night I find my temper set at a short fuse. The best thing is to say as few words as possible. Emma was in when I arrived. I noted down in the book what I had been up to. All she said was, 'I'll go and get you some tea. Perhaps you'll need coffee later.'

I went down the back to tidy up my equipment.

'Rough night, I see from the book,' said Anne, coming down from the office.

'Well, exceptional. Last week I was on duty two nights and was never called out at all,' I pointed out. 'Odd nights I have been called out once. What happened last night is not the norm.'

'Too right… good thing too!' She laughed. 'Else none of us would be able to manage. Here, let me take these away – I can sort them up front.' She grabbed some of my surgical equipment and took it away to clean.

Neil came down the back and found me tidying the rest of my kit.

'I heard you had very busy night,' he said, initiating the conversation.

'Yes, three Caesars and a womb bed out. I've never seen that before,' I replied.

'No, nor I, though I have had some busy nights as well. But Richard, next time if you are so busy for heaven's sake phone one of us, won't you?' he urged me.

'Well, I don't know,' I said.

'No – yon is ridiculous. Tell Jill from me. If you are ending up being up all night doing heavy-duty work, you must get one of us out for one call – I mean that – else you'll damage yourself.' He paused. 'I know only too well. A night like that can take a lot out of you.'

'Well…' I said.

'No well; no buts.' Neil touched the table as if in emphasis. 'Next time you must phone: no heroics. You'll be needed for another day.' I was just about to remind him about his escapade at the mart where he had been knocked out and then carried on after he came round. Then I saw his determined face.

'Okay, sure, Neil. I'll tell Jill. Next time there's a carry-on like that she'll phone either Anne or you. Promise.'

'Good,' he said. And that was the end of the matter.

Chapter Nine

Meum est propositum in taberna mori,
Ubi vina proxima morientis ori:
Tunc cantabunt laetius angelorum chori
'Sit Deus propitius huic potatori.'

I desire to end me days in tavern drinking,
May some Christian hold for me the glass when I am shrinking;
That the Cherubim may cry, when they see me sinking,
'God be merciful to a soul of this gentleman's way of thinking.'

The Archipoeta, trans. Leigh Hunt

The day had passed with no events of great moment. I finished work and dashed off to hockey practice. The all-weather pitch supplied by lottery money gave us a reasonable surface to play on. One of the joys of the Wednesday practice game was the fun of having a run around. At the end I agreed with Simon to meet him at the 'usual'. In this good humour I carried on oblivious to the reality of my situation. My poise would have evaporated had I known that the relevant quote to this particular day was: 'Unknown to Archie fate was quietly slipping the lead into the boxing glove' (PG Wodehouse).

It was dark in the street and the green lights of the automatic teller appeared bright to my eyes when I stopped by on my way to the pub. The money churned out. I quickly pocketed the notes and turned to the door situated at the corner, the entrance to the Crown bar. Every Wednesday after hockey training, Simon and I met to watch some football and quench our thirst. Football supporters of all persuasions – Celtic, Rangers, Hearts – frequented the Crown, and of course there were supporters of the local team, the Dons. Their summated expert memories went back far and wide. Gordon Banks' save from Pele in '70 was an elementary level of knowledge, while Eric Black's goals for Aberdeen in the UEFA cup were medium level. At the higher levels I hardly recognised the question, let alone the answer.

'Two pints of cider, please.' I'd arrived before Simon. Up on the screens there was only tennis to be seen. In response to my raised eyebrows the barmaid told me that for the first time for months no soccer was on air. That was a poor start. Then the phone rang. I saw the lady take the call and then come over to me.

'Simon phoned. There's a small problem at home and he's sorry but he can't make it.'

I smiled. It appeared to me that lightning or the equivalent did strike twice. Simon's absence was almost as unheard of as was the absence of football in the Crown. I gazed into the shiny depths of my pint and mused that little could get worse. Unfortunately on that point I was wrong.

'The hotelier told me I could find you here,' stated a voice behind me.

I recognised it such that the hairs started to rise on my neck. Was it possible that Mr Leasden, my old Classics master, had come to haunt me? I thought he would avoid me rather than search for me. After our meeting the previous weekend I thought we had seen enough of each other for a decade or so. For a split second it occurred to me that this could be a temporary hallucination – the effect of a combination of fatigue and drink.

I turned away from the bar to check. Sure enough the speaker had the appearance of my old Classics master. As he came towards me I clumsily touched him by the cuff. Leasden raised his hand reflexly in embarrassment. He was real. A mixture of emotions passed through me. Despite the stresses of life I could be sure I wasn't suffering from hallucinations. My brain was intact and functioning, but instead of personal psychosis I now had to deal with Leasden. The vain hope that it was a contemporary of mine imitating him for a joke had, along with my good humour, perished.

'How nice to see you,' I lied. 'You're correct: word *does* get round the town fast – so fast that I was expecting you! The pint there is for you. I remember you liked cider.' I nodded toward Simon's pint. For a second or two I had the pleasure of seeing Leasden look a little off balance. It did not last long.

'Very kind of you, Richard, don't mind if I do.' He adroitly raised himself up onto a bar stool beside me. 'You perhaps do not know that I have a niece who is vet. I was reading some of the material that comes through her office and was amazed at the drugs affair.'

I blithely wondered if his niece, contrary to his family's customary purity, had been hitting something really hard. Ketamine being too easily available, had she gone after cocaine, LSD or heroin? His next sentence woke me up from my reverie of Leasden in the witness box witnessing to the good character of his niece up on a drugs charge.

'This Competition Commission business is interesting, though I am finding it hard to apply logic and reason to it. But then I may have got it wrong; my expertise is only in Classics. Perhaps you as a practising vet could help me? I imagine they also have a veterinary surgeon or animal health professional on their commission,' he stated.

'Funnily enough, they do not have anyone with animal welfare experience in depth,' I said.

'Oh,' Leasden said. 'Oh – none at all? My word, what a peculiar way to run a ship. Still, I did see they have an accountant and economist in it. Presumably they are practised at mathematics?'

'Presumably,' I concurred. The conversation had taken a very esoteric turn. But this time I was not going to let him get the better of me, even if it meant making a fool of myself in front of the other regulars of the Crown.

'Well, as I understand it in the system detailed in paras. seventeen and eighteen, page nine, they examine if someone has more than twenty-five per cent of the market. Then, if it is so found, they deduce a monopoly may exist. How many wholesalers serve you?' he asked.

'Two, in practical terms. They fight like tigers: Dunlops and Dunwoods. Very good service is the result. Mind you, in any place in the UK you can normally only get four wholesalers. So … I get it. You're saying that logically there is bound to be one wholesaler with over twenty-five per cent of the market. I suppose that was like asking the Competition Commission to hit a barn door at two paces.'

'Precisely, but then they need to introduce new players into the market,' he advocated.

'Leasden, the margins aren't there. Only a few months ago one of them went bust. Nothing to do with unfair competition. The margins are not there, and if the prices for any reason go down significantly the profits will go down even more for the wholesalers. Don't get me wrong; I'm not trying to defend them out of self-interest. It appears from my view to be very cut-throat between them. That sounds like competition to me.' I spoke with a rather world-weary air, hoping he would change the subject

'Still, I imagine with an accountant on the Commission they've taken into consideration the bottom line.' Leasden looked at me as though once again he was in the Classics classroom asking me for the present tense of *amare*. For a split second I was about to regurgitate *amo, amas, amat*; then I gained control of myself.

'No,' I paused. 'No, you are completely wrong – that is the one thing the accountant is *not* interested in. I can almost remember the sentence in the document. It's something like this: vets "compete with each other only in the provision of total healthcare package in which the supply of POMs is bundled with the provision of services".' I looked at him head-on.

'Yes, that is in para. seven page four in the context of "gatekeepers"; I confess it is a strange use of the word "only",' Leasden continued. 'I wonder if this Commission would then say that while Premier Division football clubs engaged in many activities they *only* compete for real when eleven of their clubs players try to score more goals than eleven players from another club. What other field is of any significance?'

'Amen to that,' I said, hardly listening to him. Vainly I looked around for another topic of conversation.

'In para. ten page five, they deal with the subject of distortions, no doubt looking for efficiencies. No doubt with the economist present I imagine they have identified a way to make the system more economic and efficient,' Leasden carried on blithely. I couldn't quite make him out. I tried to curb him a bit.

'"Imagine" is the correct word, sir. I can't see how a system that used only one professional to deliver medicines and services is now more efficient and more economic when it is planned in the future in most cases to use two highly-trained professionals – a vet and a pharmacist. It really does beat me.' I took another hefty swig of my pint for consolation.

'Perhaps if one looks at their suggestions in para 24 (a) (i) and (ii) they are trying to reduce the prices of all these medicines and achieve something subtle,' he said in all seriousness.

'Or perhaps they did not realise that in place before they turned up there was something extremely subtle,' I riposted. 'The farmers with the worst management practices were subtly taxed by the costs of medicines and vet fees until they got their management correct. Thus not selling medicines at peppercorn rates stopped them relying on medicines to dig them out of their management failures. We have always wanted farm animal vaccines to be cheap; medicines are a different matter.' I regarded my nearly empty glass.

'Anyway,' I continued, 'even if the medicines do subsidise farm practice, do you not see how subtle a system of farm insurance it is? On the strength of it we give free advice all the time and any time for the animals' benefit. No one could afford the true rates of calling a vet or anyone else out late at night. This system, with no middlemen taking their cut, is the most hyperefficent way of creating a form of insurance policy for bringing out the vet at any time or place. I had my hand inside a lambing ewe at the turn of the millennium… where were you?' The drink had fired me up.

I looked to my left to see if the tennis had departed from the TV and noticed below the TV some of the regulars now looking uneasy, grimacing and sour. This sort of behaviour occurred if a man had ordered a pink gin for himself or had been rude to the fairer sex. Turning back, to my horror I found Leasden had taken out a copy of the Competition Commission document, smoothed it down on the bar and was reading aloud from it.

'In para 9 (c) on page five they state, "pricing POMs so as to subsidise, to a greater or lesser extent, professional fees…"'

'*Put it away!*' I hissed. Remarkably quickly, and without blinking, he folded it up. 'Listen,' I carried on, *sotto voce*; I decided it was time to inform him of the realities of Inverden. 'These folk here live in the real world. Not in some erudite legal, economically correct, sociological correct world where everything is examined to the last minute detail. They know about pettiness and detail ad nauseam. You may think they are intellectually inferior, but they know about the errors of pursuing righteousness to the last tithe of cumin. They know about Pharisaism and how those guys strained for a gnat with their petty Pharisee rules, and swallowed a camel by missing the Messiah when he was under their noses. They know when it comes to rules that there are only ten, I repeat *ten*, Commandments worthy of note. And they also know that Jesus shortened those Ten Commandments down to two commandments. So please do not discuss the intricacies of rules, with their implied political correctness, here. According to these folk here, "loving actions and deeds" and "legalism with pedantic detail" do not mix.' I took a breath and passed a weak grin to the other regulars.

'Fair enough,' said Leasden, apparently unmoved, and looking directly ahead of himself. 'I will stick to broad principles. Anyway, I learnt most of the points of the document off by heart as an intellectual exercise.' I did not know whether to love his quirkiness or loathe his heartless rigour. 'In the meantime, can I get you a drink? As I understand it for serious players here a nip or even a double accompanies a pint. How about it?'

'Well, fine, in that case with my pint I'll have a double Glenfarclas 105, please,' I replied. His eyebrows rose. 'A measure for measure,' I added. Leasden ordered and then quipped.

'As you like it.' Then his eyes glinted and he continued. 'With this medicines issue if you are a producer of ham, let any merchant, of Venice for example, supply all the producers' wants.'

'Oh,' I butted in, 'take a Yorkshire farmer called Henry. The fifth of his pig farms receives venetian medicine while, for Henry the fourth part I & part II, supplies will come by the two gentlemen of Verona.' I paused, and he took me up.

'And I suppose for Henry, the eighth farm could be supplied by any pharmacist Ryan, Tony, and Cleo, Pat, Randy you name it. So it appears all's well,' he baited me.

'That ends well-intentioned aims,' I carried on. 'By the destruction of the vets' first loves. Labours lost the sympathy of the profession. The comedy of errors they have created is an inept attempt to replace vets' love of animal well-being for pure commercialism.' Leasden took up the mantle.

'I can see these reviews produce within the profession the *Tempest* and even riot. Hello, that's a dark side to it.'

I cut him off. 'But for your average punter and his dog, Mr John Julius, Caesar his Alsatian, or Mrs Susan Mac, Beth her Labrador' – by now I was getting desperate – 'Mr Deaking, John his bulldog, the whole issue is much ado about nothing. The prospect of insomnia in the twelfth night of a war with Iraq is a more pressing concern these winters.' I let it hang.

'Tale or recollection to them of the calm of a midsummer night's dream will seem so very far away.' Leasden was unstoppable. 'I am sorry for you, Richard, this present government may not be for taming. Of the shrew-like character they espouse you are now well acquainted.'

'Well done,' I said. 'Your stamina beat me.'

'Oh, that's fine,' he said, in genuine humility. 'Mind you, I notice the lady serving us did not fully inform me of the price before my purchase of each of the individual items. No doubt your Glenfarclas is not cheap. *And* she did not tell me that I can purchase the same at an off licence for much less money. But then ...' he looked around the bar in a disparaging manner... 'I suppose I am paying for the whole package! A concept the Competition Commission appears not to credit. Meanwhile let us go back to principles and logic. I love logic. It appears one main thrust of the commission is for one vet A to perform the diagnosis consultation etc. and the other vet B on receipt of prescription to give out the drug?' As he offered the idea, I reflected that a terrier could not have gripped or worried at the argument as hard as Leasden.

'That's one possibility they're very keen on,' I said. 'They think B will supply medicine efficiently and cheaply, producing keen competition and efficiency.'

'But suppose A is busy handing out prescriptions, for example, to a pig farm regularly for, say, I don't know drugs, but let's try penicillin.'

'Okay.' I let him carry on.

'After the tenth tonne of medicine, is not the conscience of vet B going to be pricked? He is, after all, dishing out, no doubt with all the correct provisos, these drugs by the heap. Isn't he going to enquire at all after the well-being of the pigs?'

'Perhaps he might, certainly if he has any interest in animal welfare.'

'Do you not see, Richard, as soon as vet B even queries and says, "Is this drug helping the pigs?" he is entering a consultation process?'

'Oh, so if the pig farmer said they're not bad but have a funny skin rash, the vet might ask, "Is it diamond shaped?" – hinting at erysipelas; then that is consulting?'

'Precisely. And thus you have *one* vet consulting and handing out the medicine. In strict logic, vet B is in exactly the same position as vet A was before the changes. Previously, vet A was consulting and giving out medicines.' He looked at me.

'I suppose it could be said that this is an additional check. You know – two heads better than one,' I suggested.

'I doubt it. Do you not have a procedure for getting a second opinion?' he asked, baffled.

'Of course we do,' I said, offended. 'Furthermore, the farmer himself can ask for it, or ask the vet to get a vet lab to help.'

'Does vet A who hands out the drugs make many mistakes in prescribing? I personally doubt in relative risk terms he does. Furthermore, he would spot indifferent results very quickly. If you go back to the model of vet A and vet B, the medicine vet B hands out will now, like human medicine, have detailed instructions which vet B and the farmer will have to agree on understanding. What happens if they do not fully understand the instructions for the situation? They'll have to go back to vet A, and that is a second consultation. More cost for this consultation is incurred, never mind the costs of the client's time going from A to B. Still, it is supposed to save money.'

'Ah, but it might,' I said, ' if vet B sells it cheaply.'

'I doubt the total cost will go down much, certainly not if it is fully costed. Vet A's prescription and consultation charge will rise by almost the same amount as the profit of the drug. Thus vet B must sell the drug at almost the wholesale price and still make a profit, and ensure that the client does not have to go back to vet A for more consultation. This means one thing in logic terms.'

'What's that?' Glenfarclas required the occasional monosyllabic sentence. Besides, I had now long given up on trying to divert him.

'Vet B must act no longer as a veterinary surgeon but as a commercial agent trying to increase his turnover as much as possible. You see, there is an ethical point here. The government is changing your profession's character. Vet B becomes a type of wholesaler. I find that strange because he may well be successful, and then far more of your farm animals will end up receiving medicines than ever before. It will be quite difficult to eat anything that has not been medicated in some way. There may be great temptations present, with all those cheap medicines flowing around.'

'It's funny you say that, but the Commission are very unhappy about a bit of European legislation that says vets should have more control of those drugs going to feed animals,' I added. By now the Glenfarclas was working its magic.

'A little Janus-faced, our leaders,' observed Leasden. 'Some things of Europe they accept, others they will not. I wonder if they are huffing because the control of foot-and-mouth has been rested from your colleagues' hands and gone to Brussels?' The drink was working on him too, I thought. Still he carried on. 'There is another double irony. If they get their way, in order to remain efficient this new creation of the government – the "MRCVS wholesaler", I'll call him – will behave in certain ways, that is because he is in business. He'll aim to eliminate his opponents.'

'So-ssho?' I slurred. My brain had by now been mauled to pulp by this smiling Classics master.

'Well, after a few years there'll be only a few chains of "Wholesaling MRCVSs" pushing out very cheap medicines to all and sundry. Four chains at the most, and therefore the government will have to perform a monopoly review on them. I wonder if this is a planned way these Competition Commissions generate future work for themselves?'

'*In vino veritas?*' I suggested.

'How kind of you,' Leasden replied with alacrity. 'I'll have another for the sake of truth.' He gazed at the amber fluid when it arrived and said, 'You know the alternative quote from the same author, Pliny, is *"Vulgoque verita iam attributa vino est...* Now truth is commonly said to be in wine".'

'Yes, but for bears of little brain like myself the former is easier to recollect.' I didn't know whether Leasden was in love with his Classics or bent on a lifetime's teaching.

'I wonder if I can ask you a favour,' said Leasden, changing the subject again.

'Sure, fire away!' I was in magnanimous mood.

'I would very much like to see what veterinary practice is like,' continued Leasden. 'I wonder if you would mind if I watched you practice for a week or two or even more? It would be the equivalent of, I believe the phrase is, seeing practice; or for those into late twentieth century jargon, EMS.'

'Extramural studies,' I said. 'Though what it has to do with a wall beats me.

'I think it may be to do with the concept of studying outside the confines of the civilisation and security of the university or town. Outside *ex mura,* or extramural, outside the city walls,' he volunteered.

'Well, what an insult! We are not all barbarians here. Perhaps at this very moment I am not the best example of civilised society but my companions—' I surveyed the other regulars in the Crown— 'they are hardly in the same league as the Vandals or the Goths.'

'I am sure no insult was intended with the title EMS,' Leasden glazed over my last outburst. 'But excuse me returning to the main point, would you mind me seeing the practice with you?'

'Look, Leasden, I know I've had a few, but are you serious?' I asked him. 'I mean, if you're taking the piss, I don't mind. Really I don't. Quite a funny suggestion, actually.'

'No, I am serious. Perhaps I should have mentioned it earlier in the evening.'

'No. No, it's okay. I can make decisions, so don't worry. But I don't get it. Why?' I was mystified.

'Well, I would like to know more of what my niece is up to. I gather she is finding it quite hard. It's very difficult for me to advise her or any other members of her family unless I see what modern practice is really like. I think if I just went with her I would put her under more strain rather than help her.' He looked directly at me.

'Now that is a fair, sound and constructive reason. Very well, for the sake of the lady niece I will help you. It is not easy starting in practice, that's very true. I had to take porridge every morning to stop myself puking from nerves. I couldn't keep cereals down for the first six months. Porridge was a much better stomach stabiliser. You're still fit aren't you? Well, you appeared to be going up that hill last weekend,' I remarked.

'Yes, I am fit. Not a true Spartan, but fit enough,' he replied.

'Very well. There are one or two ground rules. Neil and I will go over them. But basically do not do anything that will make a vet look more of a chump than he has already made of himself.'

'Oh, I think I can manage that,' confirmed Leasden.

We had one more drink and then I made to get up and leave. Leasden caught me as I lurched forward.

'Steady there! I'll walk you home,' he suggested.

'No need,' I mumbled.

'Yes, there *is* a need. I will come with you.' Leasden was insistent. 'At the very least, let us leave the pub together.'

'Righto.' Very much the worse for wear, I left the pub with Leasden guiding me. The cold wind caught me. I breathed in the fresh air. My mind cleared. 'Right, I'll be fine now I'm sure.' I moved forward a couple of paces and then twisted into the wall as I lost my foothold.

I did not resist his helping me. Together we made our way down the hill and back toward my house by the river.

'Just turn in here,' I directed. Leasden helped me up the garden path and knocked at the door.

'Mrs Jones?' Leasden asked Jill as she opened the door.

'Yes? Oh, thank you. Richard, really!' she protested. 'Come in, both of you.'

'No, it's fine, thank you,' said Leasden. I glided past Jill toward a chair, which I collapsed into.

'Well, I am very grateful. He doesn't do this often. In fact the last time was when a close friend took him out and let him over-indulge himself,' Jill blathered on, embarrassed. 'That friend was a priest; I thought he would be more careful. Still, I suppose one never knows. I am grateful.'

'Well, I wouldn't hold it against the priests. I am a Classics master,' said Leaden.

'No, of course I didn't mean it like that. And I'm sure it's Richard's fault completely.' Suddenly the penny dropped. 'Are you his Latin master, Leasden?'

'Er, yes,' Leasden was taken aback by Jill's quickness.

'Well, I think a lot of you. You had your hands full with him,' she jerked her thumb to my half asleep corpse. 'At least you tried to help him.'

'Yes, it was quite hard work,' allowed Leasden.

'Still is. But that's my job. Anyway, I can't but thank you. If there's anything Richard or I can do to help do tell us. At least you got him out of the pub and back here in one piece.'

'Well, there is one thing. Could you remind him when he has come to himself that he thought he might be able to let me see practice with him? And you could remind him that I took on board his view that the person seeing practice should "not do anything that will make a vet look more of a chump than he has already made of himself"?'

'Oh,' said Jill. 'Oh, I see what you mean, Mr Leasden. In fact, I see exactly what you mean. I think I can tell you now that you and I have an understanding. Just you leave this matter to me.'

'Thank you,' said Leasden and he was gone.

'What wash that all about?' I stuttered.

'Never you mind,' was the curt reply. 'I'll tell you what you are going to do. I'll be making sure you behave properly. Mr Leasden has been good to you. Making sure you got back without causing an embarrassment. You could have been seen in the square by the bobbies. One of my colleagues might have had to prosecute you in the Sheriff's Court. You're something else! Didn't Simon try and stop you?'

'He wasn't there,' I replied lamely.

'Wasn't there!' Jill was now fuming. 'The one time a friend is not there and you go and get sotted in sorrow for yourself. Goodness!'

'It wasn't like that. Leasden asked me about the Competition Commission,' I tried to explain.

'I'm not a fool, Richard Llewellyn Jones!' She tackled me head-on. 'Except possibly when I married you; no, I take that back. It could happen to anyone. Go to bed – or do I have to carry you there?' She was aflame now.

'No, no!' I could see little point in attempting to defend myself. So we went to bed.

Chapter Ten

Venienti occurrite morbo – Meet the disease at its first stage.

Persius, AD 34–62

'Strenuous hockey training?' asked Neil as I entered the surgery. He had noted my jaded demeanour.

'No, not really. I just had a skinful. Well, not a skinful, Neil, but enough to make me happy.' I attempted to parry his knowing look, though I had to admit to myself that it was the combination of drink, Leasden, and my wife's jibes that had dulled me.

'Very wise,' concurred Neil. 'Don't want to take life too seriously. Oh, hello, Anne.'

Anne came in and proceeded to tidy up her lab coat. 'I thought for a second I saw you last night, Richard.' She was concentrating on the coat in front of her. 'There were two drunks coming down the brae. But then I caught a good sight of the old man. Very white hair. It was none of your acquaintances, Richard. Besides, the way they were going I don't think I would be seeing you here now.' She looked up at me. I smiled back.

'Ready for another day?' she said leaving the room with Neil.

'Oh, Neil!' I called him back. 'I have an acquaintance who would like to see practice. He's not a student as such, but I did promise to show him what practice is like. Is that okay by you?'

'Fine by me, Richard. I'm sure you know what you're doing. Obviously you'll have to do most of the showing round. But we'll help if necessary.' He hurried after Anne.

The phone rang and Emma called me into the office.

'It's your wife.' She handed me the phone as though it was booby-trapped.

'Richard!' she said.

'Yes, I can hear you very clearly.' She was almost shouting at me.

'I've found out that your Mr Leasden is staying at the Inverden Inn. The number is 740435. It would be a good idea if you phoned now and arranged for his watching you work.'

'I don't see the hurry,' I said dully.

'No, of course not. But it would be a good idea to do this. Just go and do it, darling. It'll be fine, I'm sure. I'll see you tonight.'

I couldn't work out from her tone of voice whether that was a threat or promise. I phoned the hotel. Leasden had already had breakfast and gone out for a walk. So I left a message suggesting he come to the practice at half past eight the next day.

By now I had come to accept the fact that he was going to see practice. It was fait accompli. I didn't mind the company: in fact it was often quite good fun to have another person around – provided they possessed common sense. That was one talent I knew he had; it was his thorough, rigorous and logical approach that scared me a little. The next few weeks with Leasden became a mishmash of memories. It was similar to working abroad in the tropics again. There the highs had been very high; the lows the nearest to hell on earth.

Prompt at eight thirty the next morning Leasden walked in and announced himself at the reception. I had briefed the girls beforehand, but even I could see that they were taken aback by his age. Leasden, however, moved his short stocky frame with ease into the office, placed his boots leggings and jacket in a corner and sat down. He waited while we settled the matters of the day. Anne came in from the lab, took a look at Leasden and stopped. She stared at me, opened her mouth closed it, tilted her head in recognition and exited.

Then suddenly we were off. Ferguson of Hillhead had phoned to say he had found a cow with staggers.

'You'd better go, Richard,' directed Neil. 'Take young Mr Leasden with you. He might as well see some action now.'

I sought out Leasden, who had disappeared, and soon we were driving through the countryside at a breakneck speed.

'Is this an urgent call?' asked Leasden, his hand gripping the door. We had climbed up a hill and were rapidly leaving Inverden behind, nestled amongst a group of hills. Leasden turned to see the town hall clock tower and the school bell tower silhouetted against the trees surrounding the town. In front of us was a short stretch of high moorland. We crossed over it at some speed and then started to descend the slopes on the other side through well cultivated farmland with many small fields and hedgerows.

'It is one of the few genuine emergencies that we have in farm animal practice,' I replied, going round a hairpin bend at speed. Leasden had a blurred and close view of the hedge. 'Surprisingly, even some calvings are not urgent calls. But this is a matter where it is important to arrive as soon as possible.'

'Why?'

'Well, the cow has very low blood magnesium. That in consequence is giving her a heart attack. The magnesium is required to ensure that the heart muscles and nerves fire in a coordinated manner.'

'Oh, so the heart is fine otherwise. It doesn't have furred up arteries or a damaged myocardium?'

'Precisely.' I could see that Leasden might make a good student. 'At the moment the heart is not going *lub-dup lub-dup* and so on. It may be doing all sorts of odd things like *dup-dup dup-lub lub-lub dulub luludup*. In fact it's often too frightening to listen to; it's much better just to treat it wisely.'

'So you just give it magnesium in the vein then?' reasoned Leasden.

'Well, no that should kill it. In fact, if you want to euthanase an animal and are short of drugs you can give it quick dose of magnesium IV, and that usually gives it a heart attack and it dies. It's a little dramatic.'

'So it is a balance,' said Leasden, trying again. 'You put in a little with some balancing agents.'

'That is correct; you'll soon see as we are almost there.'

I turned off the road and up a farm track. I saw an open gate halfway up the hedgerow on the left. Beyond it in the field I could see a vehicle and a black and white blob beside it. Although there was a break in the clouds the grass was damp due to a recent squall.

'Typical,' I said. 'Nasty weather has caused a stress to set this off, and this is the most common breed – a Hereford cross.'

The car slithered up the hill at an angle. The grass was slippery and wet. It was not a flat sward but made of small tussocks full of yellow and green blades of grass. We made our progress toward the farmer. I could see that he'd put a halter on the cow. We stopped beside his Land Rover and I ran round to the back of the car and placed some bottles, needles, flutter valves and a stethoscope on a tray. The cow was lying on her side, fitting, great and occasional breaths came from her quivering body.

'Keep your foot on the halter and to the ground,' I said to John Ferguson.

'I don't think she's going very far,' he replied. 'In fact I'm not sure she'll make it.'

'Oh, don't say that,' I said. I pushed a large needle into the jugular vein. Dark blood streamed out. This was not a good sign. The darkness indicated the lack of oxygen in the blood, and the profusion of blood suggested high venous blood pressure and therefore a failing heart. Quickly I put four millilitres of a sedative in to quieten the cow. She calmed immediately, and I could see John Ferguson thinking she had died at that moment. Then I began to race in one bottle which contained calcium phosphorus, glucose and a touch of magnesium. This was a well-known pharmaceutical mixture. I had laced some of the bottle with extra magnesium. I considered that when they were this bad it was worth the risk to give them a little magnesium directly, in spite of what I had told Leasden a minute before. If the cow survived the next thirty seconds it would have been worth the risk. She gave a couple of deep relaxed breaths.

'Hold this,' I said to Leasden. I gave him the calcium bottle and found the magnesium bottle. I set it up so that it delivered the fluid under the skin.

'I think it's finished,' said Leasden.

I took the calcium bottle from him, giving him the magnesium bottle to hold in return. Then I removed the needle, flutter valve and calcium bottle. When the magnesium had also gone in, we had finished the treatment. John Ferguson helped us move the cow round. We had to prop her up so that she'd lean against the hill and not fall over. Her head was bent back on her side; every now and the she belched. We took the halter off her and watched for a second or two. The quivering had stopped and the breathing was regular. Then we noticed she seemed to regain consciousness and look around her.

'I think that's a good sign. Best if we left her to rise in her own time,' I proposed. We could see the other cows at the end of the field coming over.

'Fine,' replied John. 'I'll check her later ... see how she goes. If she's fine tomorrow I'll take her in. I had minerals out and had just started feeding some cobs with magnesium but nothing is foolproof.'

'Aye, you're right there. If you want to discuss it more sometime, give me a phone.'

I began to pack up my stuff. When I started the car, the cow rose up and staggered away in a drunken manner.

'If she doesn't charge all over the place she'll be okay,' I told Leasden.

We drove down the field. I aimed the car at a place above the gap in the hedge where the gate was. We slid gracefully toward the gap; with a bump we left the field and regained the farm track.

'Vet Three to base,' I radioed in.

'Could you go to Alan at Easterhouse? He's brought a lamb into the farm building. He found it on its side,' requested Emma.

'Okay, I'll go there now,' I said.

'Do lambs get staggers too?' asked Leasden.

'Not lambs; ewes sometimes do. But it's more common for us to find individual ewes with low calcium. You only see lambs down with hypocalcaemia if there are many sick. This is because someone has stressed the flock by driving them or transporting them for a very long distance with little food and water,' I explained.

'So if it is an individual lamb, what could it be?' asked Leasden.

'Lying on it side paddling its legs? Well, it could be almost anything because that's what it will do just before it dies from just about every disease it can get. But no, seriously there are some common possibilities: CCN; pulpy kidney; other clostridial diseases; certain pasteurella or listeria infections ... The latter two are bacteria.'

'Ah, a bit of a mystery, then?' commented Leasden.

'Well, we're about to find out,' I said as we drove up the farm track.

Alan came out from a farm building and signalled us toward him. We went into a large airy building to find a lamb all by itself lying on well-bedded straw.

'I just got this area ready for cows. It won't stay here if it makes it,' Alan informed me. 'It was fine yesterday. They were all fine. In fact I was pleased with this group. I've wormed them and vaccinated them and they get a mineral supplement.'

'Twice?' I asked.

'The vaccine? Yes, I learnt my lesson about that. I wonder if this is CCN?' He invited an answer.

I was a circumspect. 'It could be. Let me see.' I went on to check its temperature and other clinical signs. 'Temperature is normal ... there's no sign of pneumonia ... colour is good, except a little red in this eye, but it's been lying on that side. It's blind and almost about to fit. You don't feed silage, do you?'

'Not to these,' he replied.

The lamb gave a great tremor as he spoke. I went back to the car for some thiamine. On return I pulled away some of the wool from its neck to expose the skin. Alan gave me a hand to hold it still because it had a severe tremor. Blood filled the syringe; I slowly pushed the plunger and the thiamine went in. Then I gave an injection of B vitamins into the muscle. We put the lamb's front knees under its brisket to steady it up and stop it falling over.

'I think it's CCN. You may get one or two more, Alan, so I'll leave a bottle of thiamine and a bottle of B vitamins. You can give them into the muscle – and I would do that straight away rather than wait for one of us to come to put it into the vein. Give this one an injection tomorrow if it recovers.'

'Anything I should look for?' asked Alan.

'Oh, one going off by itself, not eating, stargazing and basically foo [drunk] should make you suspicious. But mind, it can strike quickly. Have you been giving them a little bit of extra grain recently?'

'Not grain, but some cake I had to hand. It was spare so I decided to use it. It's for sheep.'

'Well, that diet change of better food may have just tipped the balance. I would throttle down on that and put a bit of straw out. Still, as I say, it usually only gets a couple.'

'He's looking better already,' noted Leasden.

'Well, Alan probably spotted him quickly,' I said. 'The quicker you treat them, if it is CCN, the better chance they have of recovery. It's most likely to be CCN, judging by this response.' The lamb was now trying to rise.

'I'll go and make a pen for him now,' said Alan.

'While you're doing that, Leasden and I will wander through the field to see if there are any others. It's the field opposite, isn't it?' I asked.

'No, the one next to it, sloping down the hill. There are mainly wee Cheviot crosses I got from up north,' said Alan.

Leasden and I went out of the building and found the gate. We climbed over and started to walk down the field. It was surrounded by hedgerows and was about forty acres in size. The lambs were spread all over the field, which had a good covering of grass. We skirted round the edge watching the sheep. Nearly all had their heads down, grazing. Once at the bottom of the field we walked up the centre. We passed by the low feed troughs, which were empty except for a few pieces of cake. He had been too generous to them. How ironic, I thought. One or two lambs ran away from us. All appeared normal.

'See anything?' I asked Leasden.

'No, nothing with fits, no stargazing, all eating,' he replied. I admired his methodical approach. He was obviously trying to take this seeing practice seriously. We returned to the top and told Alan, who was waiting by the gate. He said he hadn't spotted any others.

Leasden and I found a tap to clean our boots under and then we left.

'CCN stands for what?' asked Leasden when we were back in the car.

'Cerebrocortical necrosis,' I replied.

'Ah, death of the outer edge of the brain,' Leasden reasoned.

'The benefits of a classical education,' I observed.

'Yes, but it still doesn't tell me how the disease occurred,' he said, pursuing the matter.

'You're right there. In fact it's quite interesting and shows how peculiar nature can be. They don't know the full story, but so far as they can work it out, the change in the diet causes a group of gram positive bugs to proliferate in the rumen. This slows the rumen down a bit but more importantly some of these bugs produce thiaminases. These are enzymes that destroy thiamine. Simply put, at short notice the animal becomes catastrophically low in thiamine. Some of the brain cells and heart cells need thiamine. They start dying off at quite a rate. Some say millions of cells in the brain are dying as you look at the animal. Perhaps that's a little dramatic. Anyway, the brain also swells. Hence all those brain-associated symptoms like drunkness and blindness are most fitting.'

'And luckily for you a good shot of thiamine quickly given cures them,' interrupted Leasden.

'Most of them,' I corrected him. 'Some don't come right because they're not CCN, and others because they're too severe or have been sick for too long to stand a chance.'

'Well, so far my first two animals have been lying on their sides quivering,' said Leasden.

'There will be at third,' I murmured.

'What did you say?' asked Leasden

'Nothing. Just rural superstition. Vet Three to base?' I radioed in.

'Vet Three can you go to Westerhouse? They have a calf with scour that isn't responding to treatment,' June requested.

'Right, I'll go there now,' I decided. I stopped the car, checked around me and then turned back.

We arrived at Westerhouse to be greeted by the grieve. He showed us the calf, which was in a small pen made of lorry pallets. There was a lot of straw underneath it. It was only just able to rise. I quizzed the grieve. The calf was a week old and had been born to an heifer. She had not been vaccinated before calving. This meant the heifer's colostrum and milk possessed few antibodies against the common causes of diarrhoea. It wasn't a big surprise to find the calf ailing. I looked at it. They always are a sorry sight at this stage: its eyes were slightly sunk in its sockets; its coat stared at me: it was no longer shiny and sleek; its flanks were 'clapped in'. I nipped over a pallet and took its temperature. Foul yellow-white froth and diarrhoea came out with the thermometer. The temperature was just normal. Any lower and the calf's life expectancy would be poor. The skin 'tented' when I pinched it instead of snapping back to its normal position. The heart was fortunately beating at a regular rate. Its eye mucous membranes were red, which suggested acidosis. The inside of the mouth was cold and it had a poor sucking reflex.

'I'll give it a drip and one or two other things,' I said, and turned to the car. Leasden watched over my shoulder as I prepared the drip we had perfected in the practice. It was an hypertonic solution which, amazingly, could be given to a calf very quickly in a matter of a few minutes. This coupled with some powerful supportive medicines cured over half the calves that farmers had given up on because their fluid therapy was not succeeding.

We returned to the calf. The grieve and I sat the calf down and tilted its neck to one side. Then he sat behind it and steadied its head to make sure it couldn't move around while we gave it the drip. I clipped up the requisite part of the neck. Then I put my thumb against the neck and emptied and filled the jugular vein in the jugular groove a couple of times. This was to make certain I knew exactly where it was. At the top of the jugular I put in a short wide-bored needle. It hit the vein as the blood 'flashed back' into the syringe. I pressed the plunger and so gave some potent anti-inflammatory to the calf. Then I carefully removed the syringe from the needle. Blood flowed from the end. Leasden passed me the tube from the drip, which I fixed onto the needle. I let it flow in. All the time I checked the rate of flow of the solution into the calf and examined the skin near the needle closely. Any swelling would mean we had 'blown' the vein and would have to start again. Equally well, the rate of flow often slowed down if the needle exited the jugular.

Halfway through the calf gave a lurch. The needle wobbled and we lost it from the jugular. Undeterred, I took the needle out, married it up to a syringe and found the jugular a few inches further down the groove. It was now easy to find because the first part of the drip had already raised the venous blood pressure. We managed to complete the administration. I handed back the tubes and needles to Leasden, who was standing just outside the pen.

He lowered his hand which had been holding the drip bottle and replaced all the pieces in a tray.

The grieve and I then put a stomach tube in the calf and gave it two litres of fluids. The calf seemed a bit brighter when we left. I gave the grieve instructions on what to do next. Leasden and I found a tap and hose. I told him to disinfect with care as the bugs for calf diarrhoea are easily carried from farm to farm.

'Well, that was standing and not quivering,' I told him.

'Yes. Thought a little variety would come in soon.'

Our next visit was to a couple of calves with pneumonia. It looked as though we'd be able to head back for an early lunch. I radioed in.

'Can you go to Chris Remmington, Amblefield? One of his horses' legs is swollen again,' June advised me.

'Righto,' I said. 'Now we're going to see a horse. Captain Remmington is a pilot and perhaps the most reasonable horse owner I have ever known.'

'Oh!' Leasden appeared baffled. 'What is it likely to be?'

'It is all a bit odd, but he has three nice mature grey horses and every now and then one of their legs blows up. The technical term must be lymphadenitis. What we've found out is by going to them quickly and treating them with antibiotics and steroids in the vein they are usually right the next day. Conversely, we have found if you delay it twelve hours or so because you think there's no urgency, then it becomes difficult to treat. The horse is fine – eating and so on – but that is deceptive.' I tried to give him some background.

'So speed is the essence?'

'Well, no need to delay,' I replied.

A quarter of an hour later we were there. I got out.

'This horse has done it again. He always messes things up. He knew I had a lunch date. So what does he do but go and get this again,' said the owner. He was smart, fit and obviously ready for non-equine activities. The only compromise to the horse matter was a pair of wellingtons.

'Well, we'll try and be quick. If I remember aright last time, he did this just before you were going on holiday to the States.'

'Exactly! Choose an inconvenient moment and he will,' agreed Chris Remmington.

By now we were walking across the field toward the small house for the horses. Leasden followed in our wake through the thick grass. Half in and half out of their little shelter stood the two Highlanders. They were large handsome animals with big solid hooves. We stopped by the gate five yards from them and it was obvious that one had a grossly swollen leg in a sector arising from the fetlock and going up to the hock. I checked the horse. There was little untoward. Chris Remmington held his head while I clipped away the very shaggy winter coat. I gave him the medicines I had given a few times before.

'It's about once every eight months, isn't it?' asked Chris Remmington.

'Something like that,' I concurred. 'Of course, we could investigate it further, though that will cost a pretty penny and I'm not sure it's worth it – particularly as the old boy has an odd melanoma. This condition is probably lymphadenitis.'

Horses with grey colouration were notorious for developing melanomas. Fortunately, in Highlanders they were usually not rapidly lethal. The same growth in a dog or human being was potentially lethal if no treatment was started quickly. Even then, with dogs the majority die soon after diagnosis.

'Agh, we will see. They seem happy enough. Wouldn't you agree?' said Chris.

'I think so. Anyway, if it seems to be getting out of hand we can do more. But I don't mind our present arrangement … provided it doesn't cramp your social life too much,' I teased him.

'Cheeky! Mine is nothing compared to your colleague and senior partner's,' he laughed.

'Last time you told me you were flying around the Highlands getting a close view of Glen Bogal and Loch Ness and so on,' I ventured.

'Ah, that is *work*, showing people the Highlands from a different perspective,' he countered.

'You don't enjoy it?'

'Oh, I enjoy it. The views are terrific. Don't get me wrong, but it's still work. The only thing I feel guilty about is showing people groups of deer on the hill. The shooters are not very good at broadcasting where they're hunting. So we may disturb some deer just as someone is completing a three-hour stalk and about to shoot. That could annoy them,' he told us.

'That's odd,' I said.

'Well, I know from my service contacts that information about stalking is given to the RAF, but the shooters don't give it to civilian people, or they're not so efficient. On RAF maps they'll have areas marked off for a day. In fact they have bits of plastic shaped in those zones which they stick on the map, saves on the drawing of complex boundaries again and again. Oh, is that the time?' He looked at his watch.

'We must go too. Nice to see you. Here's the medicine for the next three days. One whole paste a day for three days.' I handed him three enormous blunt-ended syringes. They contained an antibiotic paste which he would give to the horse by mouth. We left at speed.

As we came round a corner we saw a car had stopped about a hundred yards ahead of us. I slowed down. The driver was out. He was gazing at something in the deep grass just off the road. I stopped beyond him and got out. I noticed a headlight on the car was smashed.

'Can you help me?' said the driver. 'I don't know what to do. A deer jumped out and I slowed down a bit but then a second one jumped out right in front of me. There was a terrific *thunk* and the body went flying into the verge here. He has never got up. It only happened a few seconds before you came.' The deer was lying on its side, shaking. Bloody froth was coming out of its nose. A hind leg was badly shattered.

'I'll get something from the car to help,' I said, as they stood by. 'I knew there would be a third,' I muttered as I ran to my car and opened the boot. I grabbed a bottle of euthanasia fluid, a syringe and a needle. I trotted back to the others.

'I think he's gone,' said the driver. Sure enough, the deer was motionless. I stood holding the needle and syringe in my open hands: there was no need for them now. 'I don't know what to do. I haven't got any room for it in my car. Can you dispose of it?' the driver asked plaintively. Suddenly I woke up from my reverie. I had been staring at the beautiful shape of the deer's head.

'Dispose of it?' I blurted out. 'Sure, I can do that. I'm a vet. We often have to dispose of things like this. You leave it to me. I have a bag in my car. You'll probably want to go and get your car fixed.'

'Thanks, thanks a lot,' said the driver. 'Are you sure that'll be okay?'

'Yes, just leave it to me,' I replied.

The driver quickly got back into his car. I could see that he was still somewhat upset and only wanted to do one thing: leave the accident scene. He shot away. All went quiet. I hadn't moved. The road stretched silent and straight in front of us. Tall conifers on either side lent an eerie feel to the moment. Leasden moved first.

'Well, your bag?'

'Blanket, actually,' I told him, returning in a brisk walk to my car.

'What are you going to do with it?'

'Eat it, of course,' I said curtly. 'We are omnivores. You taught me Latin: *omnis vorare*. *Omnis* means all or everything, and that includes deer. *Vorare* – to swallow or devour. So that is what I am, my dear teacher. Anyway, we'll hang it at the back of the surgery for a few days. Can you give me a hand, please.'

With remarkable speed we had it wrapped up and in the boot. No one had passed by or seen us.

'Vet Three to base,' I radioed.

'Nothing new,' said June.

'June, can you open the back in a few minutes? I have something to deliver,' I said in a deadpan voice.

'Is it edible?' she asked.

'Yes.'

'Oh, I think I know what to prepare. I'll have a wordy with Anne. See you in five minutes.'

'Fine,' I said.

When we arrived at the back of the surgery we found Anne waiting for us. She was wearing protective overalls. She admired our offering. We took it inside. She deftly tied a rope to the deer's hock and raised it up. It hung from one of the rafters. She grabbed a knife.

'I'll take out the innards,' she said. 'It'll hang a bit better, in my opinion. Sometimes they can rot a bit too quick.'

I left them too it. Leasden, under Anne's instruction, held bags which she filled.

'These are the stomachs coming out now,' she described. 'Not squeamish are you?'

'Not really,' answered Leasden.

'I did Classics as well, you know,' she volunteered. 'I think I enjoyed it more than Richard. It certainly helped me with grammar in all other languages.'

'Yes, it does have many uses.' Leasden was not to be drawn.

'Kidneys,' explained Anne, pulling them out and plopping them into the bag which Leasden held open.

'Quite.'

'I sometimes thought my Classics master missed a trick or two. I remember how important the Romans thought the sacrificial poultry were. We kept on hearing about people looking into the entrails of a hen. For people like me who also like biology, the Classics master should have done a practical. It would've been fascinating.'

'What?'

'Well, they should have had a practical on the intestines of poultry. What upset the Roman priests and what they thought were good signs. You know, many children are pretty bloodthirsty. Don't you think?'

'Yes, I suppose many are. But do you think it would be too traumatic?' asked Leaden

'For some boys, maybe,' said Anne, concentrating hard. She plunged her hand deep into the body of the deer and brought out the heart. It was steaming. 'But most girls are solid-hearted, if you see what I mean.' She slowly put the heart into the bag. 'Not cold-hearted, but constant and not lily-livered.'

'You may have a point.' Leasden appeared unconvinced.

'That's the lungs. We're done. Lunch?' Anne was the complete calm professional.

'Yes. I'll just clean my hands … Excuse me asking, but Neil is, how would you say, quite masculine. How did he employ a lady vet like you for mixed farm work?' asked Leasden.

'How do you mean?' Anne was suspicious.

'Well, you're not in appearance a tomboy or such. You are

feminine. Yet Neil gives the appearance that this is a male preserve,' explained Leasden.

'Ah, I see what you're getting at!' Anne laughed. 'That's easy. I'd already done farmwork and was able to do it. You also forget that Neil is interested ultimately in excellence or the best.'

'So you were the best of the applicants?'

'Seems so, that's why he employed me.' Anne dried her hands.

'I only ask because I have a niece who is in mixed farm practice and she's finding it hard. Would that be likely?'

'Very likely,' Anne agreed. 'It's much harder for a woman to be really and truly accepted on equal terms on farms, particularly if you try to maintain some feminine demeanour. You have to build up a good track record, and that's hard. There are always the snide remarks about lack of power. Right enough, you do have to build a bit of strength up top. But even if you ask Richard he'll admit that he was weak in the shoulders to start with. Then you have the sex difference.'

'What do you mean?' asked Leasden.

'Oh, you turn up to calvings where you have to go right inside the cow to find the feet and correct the head. Some farmers like to suggest you strip off to the waist like the boys. I can do without that; I must admit it's not as bad as it used to be. But if you are lacking in confidence it hardly helps.'

'Are you?' Leasden expressed doubt.

'Of course not. But I have got to go close, right inside it. So I have ended up with some very dirty clothes which came inside the cow with me.'

'That's a touch unfair.'

'Well, you take the rough with the smooth. Also, for example, if there is a farm animal with something wrong with its penis you'll find farmers not very keen on giving me detailed description. That is so even when I'm standing right next to the beast. For many it's a type of mental block. They'll tell Neil and Richard everything and probably add a joke to it.'

'Difficult, isn't it?'

'Yes, I suppose so. But my word of advice to your niece is to keep at it and realise that it just takes longer to gain acceptance. If she can do the job she can succeed. Even Neil and Richard have disasters now and then, you know.'

'Well, thank you for advice. I am grateful.'

'Oh, it's okay. If your niece wants a chat and if you think that would help you can give her my phone number,' Anne suggested. 'By the way, a few nights ago was it you with Richard moving down the lane toward his house? I'd never seen anything like that before.'

'The answer is yes. And it was me, and yes; I doubt you will see anything like that again. Can we leave it at that,' replied Leasden.

'Oh, for certain. We all have private lives to lead. Mind you, I hope Richard realises that the street from the Crown to his house is hardly private.'

'Oh, I think Jill has made him aware of that.'

'Has she really?' Anne laughed. 'Well, she'll straighten him out. When she starts to prosecute, watch out!'

They moved out and up to the reception.

'All done?' asked June turning round from the computer. 'I guess it's time for lunch.'

They all went their separate ways, leaving Emma who had just come in to man the phones.

Chapter Eleven

I see the rural virtues leave the land.

Oliver Goldsmith, 1730–1774

At two p.m. I returned to find Anne and Leasden in conversation.

'I didn't realise you had a more illustrious surname,' said Anne.

'Really?' I replied, deadpan.

'Yes, I sneaked it out of your colleague here.' She nodded to Leasden. 'While we were chatting, I asked the surname of your Aunt Sarah. He let slip it was Llewellyn-Jones. The I twigged it must be your family name.'

'I suppose it's a bit of a mouthful,' I replied, 'so we have stuck to Jones. It's simpler. In fact we're not pure Welsh, quite the opposite. I know of Scottish, Irish and Yorkshire blood in our family. So we are the genuine British hybrid.'

'Mongrel vigour?' teased Anne.

'As you say, Anne,' I carried on. 'I suppose I'm not a pure bred like you, with a surname Trumpington.'

'Touché!' She smiled. 'There are one or two calls this afternoon.'

'Yes,' Emma joined in. 'Richard, could you see Mrs Simms? It's a dog booster. Then could you go to Gall, Dykestone. They have a pony which is a little dull and lame. After that White, Broomhill. He has two or three calves to castrate. Anne can do the rest of the surgery; some of the folk are for her. The two farms are close to each other, aren't they?'

'Oh, yes, they are,' I concurred. 'They're slap bang in the middle of the Glacks of Garrough.'

'The Glacks of Garrough?' asked Leasden.

'Yes,' I added. 'It's a peculiar place. A whole series of crofts in a small glen. It's extraordinary, almost a time warp. Either it's the people in it or it attracts a certain type of less forward thinking person. On top of that there's always some petty criminal activity going on.'

'Such as?' Leasden was interested.

'The burn at the bottom of the glen carries salmon. Poachers are often at it, and the bobbies have a go at getting them. It's almost a local sport. Then on the odd occasion some people have attempted to grow a bit of marijuana under cloches there. Once again, via an imaginative gossip network, the police were alerted. None of it was big-time stuff. It's hard to believe, but some of the farms only received electricity for the first time about ten to fifteen years ago. It's certainly another world there. Anyway, we'd better see Mrs Simms.'

Leasden and I went into the consulting room.

'Hello, Mrs Simms! Booster time is it?' I started my queries.

'It certainly is,' responded the lady. 'Come on, Major, up you get. One leap!' She patted the tabletop. In response the back Labrador jumped up on the table and sat there wagging his tail. He fixed his eye on Mrs Simms. I admired him. It's no surprise many vets favour black Labradors; they are a delight to deal with. Major sat still while I examined him. He was about two to three years old, and fit.

'He's by himself now of course,' said Mrs Simms. 'Bobby, our other, was put down a few months ago by Neil. He had had a good life. Anyway, we'll soon be getting a replacement for Bobby.' I saw Major's ears prick up at the mention of the name.

'Yes, I heard about that,' I said. 'Well, anyway, today I'll just give him this injection. It is not the full booster. He got that last year. We alter them a bit as they get older.'

'Yes, I saw something in the press about that.' Mrs Simms frowned a bit. 'It seems very complex.'

'It is quite complex, and changing all the time.' I wanted to help her. 'What I can tell you is that we've not had any major dog disease problems in this area for years. If we do have a disease come here, then phone us, and we can look at Major's records and double-check to see that he's had a recent booster relevant to the disease or that at least his cover is sufficient.' While I said that I injected Major under the scruff.

'I think we could weigh him,' I suggested.

At her command Major jumped down and went to the scales.

'Twenty-seven kilos; that's fine.' I noted it down. 'Has he been wormed recently?'

'Oh yes. I do that every three months. I'm up to date on that, thank you,' she replied.

'Fine. Well, we'll see you in a year's time,' I said, handing back the card.

'Oh, it might be sooner,' Mrs Simms grinned. 'It may be with a puppy. We've put out some feelers.' She left to settle up with the girls.

'We'd better go to the Glacks now,' I told Leasden.

I went down the back to pick up some equipment for the horses. Then we drove away out of the ring of hills round Inverden and down into the next large glen. As we drove along the bottom of this glen a broad low gap appeared on our right. This was the Glacks of Glarrough. It was a long, shallow glen and you could see along its length for miles. Although there was pasture on the right of the burn, only two of the crofts were on that side. These two crofts could only be reached by fording the burn by foot or with a tractor. Then one continued along the gravel tracks to the farm buildings. The remaining crofts were reachable by a thin, curvaceous metalled road. High up the left side of the glen was 'the high road'. This was a single-file gravel track which also connected with all the crofts by farm tracks. Though it was designed for bicycles, walkers and beasts, on occasion a drunk driver would exit the glen along this track and in the process damage his car. By common consent tractors were rarely found on this track, and if they did encounter anything the common law was the tractor had to reverse all the way back to the next passing place. This was one reason few tractors used it.

'Here we go,' I muttered to Leasden. We drove up the Glacks. All the crofts appeared neat but windswept. Some farms still baled hay in an old-fashioned way in great heaps with covers on top. All over the fields you could see a great variety of livestock. Not a great number, but a few well spaced out sheep, goats, horses and cattle were visible. Inside some of the buildings there would certainly be an odd pig or two.

We drove up a track to a small croft. There were signs that builders were carrying out improvements. A few contiguous low farm buildings stood opposite the house. Together they formed a small court. On the ground there was a mixture of mud with rubble underneath. I remembered Mrs Gall had come up from England last year. Rumour had it that she had had a messy divorce but had at least obtained a large amount of capital and cash. Now she and her two daughters were trying to make a new life and forget the traumatic past. I wondered whether they would succeed in the task of making a new life but fail in dealing with the trauma of the new and challenging stresses here. They were probably ill equipped to cope with these. So many 'white settlers' – as the locals called them – only lasted two to three years and then decided to return to the country and people they knew. So often they had decided on a place in the north on the strength of a summer visit and their meeting local folk who were anxious to please. I knew no place on earth was Utopia. It was a pity so many still held onto such dreams.

'I made a mistake,' said Mrs Gall, coming out of the house.

Leasden, she and I formed a triumvirate on the edge of the mud and rubble. Her hair, blouse and jumper were all very neat. However her jeans and wellies were smattered in mud and had seen better days. I wondered whether as the months passed the state of unkemptness would progress upwards to the head.

'I felt a touch sorry for him yesterday. It was beastly weather. So I gave him a handful of barley. I really mean a handful,' she continued.

'Does he often get barley?' I asked.

'No, not at all,' she responded. 'Well, it's flying from him now. Or it was this morning. It's a little firmer now.'

'Well, you've probably purged him,' I observed. 'Has he showed any signs of colic?'

'Mercifully, no. Anyway, come here. I've got him in here.' We followed her into the low building. 'Your nurse Emma mentioned something about soft bedding so I got some shavings and have put a heap in, as you can see.'

We bent down as we entered through the low doorway. Inside we saw the small chestnut pony. He was obviously uncomfortable standing up, shifting his weight from foot to foot. Mrs Gall held him while I took his temperature and checked his pulse. Fortunately both were not significantly raised. I examined the colour of his mucous membranes; they were a little injected. Using my stethoscope I could hear the intestines were moving at a fair rate. After checking a couple of other parameters I moved to the important area: the hooves. Each hoof felt a little warm; I had felt hotter. There was also a distinct pulse palpable in the vessels below the fetlocks. I had to hand some hoof testers. A small amount of pressure caused the pony to flinch. When I pushed at the coronary band just above the hoof, the pony also resented it.

'What's his name?' I asked.

'He's called Brigadier,' replied Mrs Gall, 'or Brig for short; other times he's called something unprintable.' She gave a short laugh. 'He's not a bad boy, really, just occasionally headstrong.'

'Well, in my opinion Brig has laminitis right enough,' I told her. 'I've seen better cases and I've seen worse. At least he's not a big horse with large plate-like hooves: the pedal bone can drop through those with ease. And his temp and pulse are not too bad. However, he's very uncomfortable in his feet.'

'Yes, I can see that,' she said. 'The bone can go through the sole if it separates from the hoof, isn't that it?' I noticed that nowadays many owners had a good grasp of basic horse medicine.

'Yup,' I said. 'So we'll do a variety of things. We'll put some styrofoam shoes on his feet. You'll have to give me hand, I'm afraid. How's your back? I need each foot to be held while I put this shoe on with sticky tape.'

'Oh, not too bad,' she said.

'Then I'll give him a shot of bute in the vein and we'll give him a sedative ACP. Some people think it makes little difference but it's worth a try, I think, in his case. Those two will take away a lot of pain and calm him a bit. Next I'll advise you on feeding. Right now he is to be on hay and water. To be honest, Anne is our expert at feeding laminitic horses, so I'll have a word with her. One of us will come back tomorrow and put on another set of these styrofoam shoes. I'll just get my stuff. Can you give me a hand?' I asked Leasden. We walked back to the car.

'Like *Blue Peter*,' I said to Leasden, handing him the box of styrofoam shoes, 'these I made before. I wondered if this case was going to be laminitis, even though it's the wrong time of year. It's usually due to a change of pasture, but then poor Mrs Gall shouldn't have given old Brig some barley. She's lucky; it could have been much worse.'

At that moment a pale teenager came in the close carrying a satchel.

'You must be the vet. Is Brig going to be alright?'

'I hope so,' I answered. 'Why not come and give us a hand?'

'I'll just change my shoes,' she said, rushing off.

Leasden and I returned to the pony with all our pieces.

'That sounded like my daughter,' observed Mrs Gall. 'She must have skipped the last lesson and got a ride back. Brig means a lot to her.'

'Well, don't worry, hopefully this'll do the trick.'

I showed her the styrofoam blocks shaped like the soles of a hoof. I demonstrated how we would have to place each block under the hoof. The end result would be the pony would be walking on platform soles. These he would crush down in the next twenty-four hours. The foot would be protected from the worst ravages of laminitis by the well-balanced support the platforms gave the foot.

Mrs Gall bent down and lifted the first foot. I positioned myself to apply the first block. The daughter came in and took the control of the head collar from Leasden. He moved away and found an empty space in one of the wooden troughs against the wall. He gave it a cursory wipe and sat down with his short legs dangling down. It was not unlike having a large bird observe our endeavours. Both Mrs Gall and I were bent down close to the hoof. Our heads almost met but we could not see each other. We were both concentrating our eyes on the hoof and trying to forestall the slight movements of the pony. A slight sweat broke out on both of us as we worked away. In circumstances such as this a strange communion commences in the closed little world around the foot. We could almost whisper into each other's ears.

'That's it, steady a little. Are you okay? It's not too heavy for you?' I asked.

'No, I am fine. He's a weight but I can manage. Have you got enough tape on that side?'

'Yes, I see what you mean,' I concurred. 'I'll put a bit more on there. Have I got enough at the front?'

'Let me see...' She lowered her head and peered round. 'Yes, that's fine.'

By the second hoof we did not need to speak about the shoe and the tape. We knew exactly what we were doing. The subject matter wandered.

'How are you managing now that you've been up six months or more?' I asked.

'Oh, okay,' Mrs Gall confided. 'I do find it a bit lonely. But then I did want to get away from it all a bit. Fortunately, Karen and Lucy – my girls – have made good friends, so I am pleased about that. That is the most important to me.'

'Yes. I know it can be tricky,' I agreed, 'but if you get about a bit you'll meet some folk almost as nice as you, if you see what I mean.'

'Oh, I know what you're saying,' she sniggered. 'I have to admit that I do go out to church, of all places. I went a bit before I came up about twice a year. I suppose I have a faith.'

'That's good. I can recommend you do that. I go to a kirk as well. It's not earth-shattering but I think it's important.'

'I feel there's some sort of presence, which I'm going to learn more of,' added Mrs Gall. 'But I also admit I go because I'm lonely a bit and need to meet some people.'

'Good, that's what church is for as far as I'm concerned: to worship, feel His Presence and to meet people. I do find the term "fellowship" a bit intense, but then I'm a public school boy.'

'I guessed as much.' She spoke through tight clenched teeth, for the leg was now weighing on her. 'You can't hide it. However hard you try. Even coming up to these wastes doesn't hide it.' It was my turn to snigger. She carried on. 'The church is full of different people. Sometimes I don't know if I belong or not.'

'Ah, but that's just the point,' I muttered. Sweat was coming down and misting my glasses. 'The church is designed for the dregs, the no hopers and for those who know that despite appearances everyone has a piece of them that is very rotten. Don't you think?'

'Oh, I can go along with that,' she said. 'After my divorce I learnt one thing clearly: we are, and I include myself in this, a very sorry lot when it comes to any kindness of heart. There's a streak of malevolence in us that's frightening. I suppose we keep it under control a bit. But goodness! After all the lawyers, ex-spouses, ex-in-laws and other relatives I've had to deal with, I'm certain I need time to think.'

'I'm married to a lawyer,' I said. She moved. 'No need to apologise. I'm not too impressed with them, to be honest. Okay, I'm not as white as drifted snow, but lawyers are different; many do possess "a touch of the night" about them. Perhaps it's not their fault; maybe it's the job.'

'Maybe more of them should be in church,' said Mrs Gall, as she and I placed one foot slowly down on the ground.

Brig moved as he tried to come to terms with the fact that the foot was now an inch and a half higher and with a comfortable soft cushion. We went on to the next foot.

'Well, I feel I can be comfortable in a church on two grounds. One it was designed for me and others. I have a wicked mind,' I said. She tut-tut-tutted. 'No, no, I do. Ask my lawyer wife,' I continued, 'she has enough evidence. It is mainly selfishness on my part. The other comfort is the knowledge that the first person into heaven with Our Lord was a convicted murderer. A brigand, not a rotarian, not a vet, not a lawyer nor a crofter. So if the criminal got in, then there's hope for us all; you, me.'

I stood up. 'Your daughters, and also Mr Leasden here, all stand a chance. Even hope for a Classics master, you know.' I looked intently at him. He smiled back to me.

We stood back and looked at our handiwork. It was noticeable that Brig was more comfortable on his feet. The hooves were all covered with black shiny tape which went almost up to the fetlocks. He was not shifting his weight so much. I could see hope coming into the daughter's expression. I instructed them to put more soft shavings in and arranged a time the next day to change and add more styrofoam blocks. We left them with some sachets of phenylbutazone to be given in the feed the next morning.

'Vet Three to base, I'm going on to White's now. Is Anne there?'

'No, she's had to go out to a calving,' replied June. 'Anything in particular?'

'Yes, June. Could you make a note in the book that I need to speak with her about feeding Brig, Mrs Gall's laminitic pony? Also can you make a note that one of us has to go back tomorrow to put another set of styrofoam shoes on the pony? Also can you order another set of styrofoam shoes, small size, from either Dunlops or Dunwoods? Either will do.'

'Small size?'

'That's right. If you're worried about the description, go down the back and get one of the boxes of the other sizes. They all have the same manufacturer's name.'

'Fine that,' responded June. 'In the meantime I have to tell you Anne had to rush away to a calving so she asked a man to come back at four to four thirty to see you. He has some tropical animal to look at. Anne thought it was more your line of country; besides, she was in a rush and this man said he could wait.'

'What type?' I asked.

'Dinna ken,' replied June. 'It was in a styrofoam box for insulation. I didn't want to know. It's for you not me.'

'Righto. Well, we're going to White's now.'

'Do you get many tropical animals to treat?' asked Leasden. 'Do they always push them in your direction if they do?'

'No we don't get many,' I said curtly. 'It's a little odd. My course was mainly to do with tropical diseases and how they affect animals such as Zebu cattle, goats, pigs, horse, mules et cetera. Even in the small animal clinics abroad, it was mainly dogs, cats and parrots I saw. Plus the odd piglet. Most of the local folk didn't have time or energy for the exotics. Anyway, now they think I'm the expert. Well, I just use general principles and get good advice.'

'So you haven't done much with exotics or dangerous animals?'

'Well, I've done a bit but that's more by accident than design. I've handled a tiger, but that was a cub. When I had to deal with some adults in a zoo I kept well out of their reach. I've handled an adult lion but then I made sure it was unconscious before I touched it. I've treated a jaguar. All I did then was put a wormer in the feed. I did handle an adult cougar; you can domesticate them. That was good fun, I try to avoid venomous snakes and I've had to deal with a few. The king cobra, the fer de lance, and the spitting cobra are ones I'd rather I hadn't had to deal with. The fer de lance will actually go for you with no provocation. I once had to run away from one. Luckily I have never to my knowledge been near a mamba. I did study the subject of snakes for a while but then decided it was really too dangerous. At some point one will be troubled by the "familiarity breeds contempt" problem. Surprisingly, I don't rate them the most dangerous group of animals. There's another group I am very careful of.'

'Really?' Leasden prompted me.

'Yes, primates – including man – are the ones to watch. In the jungle it is man or related primates who can be dangerous and must be treated with respect. The majority of the other mammals and animals will run away from you. Chimps are very dangerous. All primates are intelligent, quick, and have a ferocious bite. I can only remember two cases I had to handle. One I was very lucky with. I had taken the history and just come to the point where I had to handle the little horror. Then I noticed his skin was crawling and actually moving with lice. He was covered with a major infestation. I stopped my clinical examination there and then, instructed the keeper how to treat the monkey and left.'

'So you don't like primates?'

'There was one exception I slept with a primate a few times. Josh. He was okay.' I paused but Leasden didn't move.

'He was a very young orang-utan. His mother had been shot, and my men arrested the smuggler. So I looked after him for a few days while the zoo got their premises and keeper ready for him. We used to change his nappy and so on; it was just like having a baby. Take him for short walks, bottle-feed him and so on. I kept him warm at night. It was peculiar. I became very broody. I believe it's a recognised syndrome.'

'Strange, I can't see you becoming broody,' remarked Leasden.

'No, it was weird,' I said. 'Eventually my boss, the senior vet, and the zoo came to take Josh away to his new quarters. I was heartbroken; so was my wife and the maid, Juliet. Not a dry eye in the house for two days. Well, that's history … here we go. I'd keep your eyes peeled here.'

We had moved to a different section of the Glacks of Garrough. I drove the car down a short, straight farm track. The middle of the car brushed against the grass in the centre of the track. In front of us were a series of low, ancient granite farm buildings. Just behind them was one more modern farm building a little taller than the rest. The chimneys on the house were not straight and the odd tile was loose. A low hedge close to the building hid the state of the brickwork. The windows were present but appeared from our close view to be opaque with grime. I turned the car round into the close. A tall lanky man stood there holding a bucket of warm water in one hand and soap and towel in the other. Mr White was a man of tradition. This was one I appreciated.

'Afternoon,' he said. 'Not bad, is it?'

'No, not bad at all,' I said. Leasden looked up at the light grey sky in surprise; but this was good weather for the time of day and the season.

'I've just got three to cut,' said Mr White. 'I put horn paste on them when they were born and it seems to have worked. If you like you can check them.'

We moved into the byre to see five calves tied up along one wall. On the other side stood two cows. Mr White was into some form of multiple suckling.

'Well, they're handy like that,' I said. 'If you can jam them against the wall one by one I'll cut them for you.'

'Right. I thought you and I would manage, so I didn't want to hinder Jimmy by asking him over for a hand.' Jimmy was his neighbour. They often helped each other out.

Mr White pinned a calf against the wall. I bent down behind it. I took a scalpel out from the bucket into which I had placed disinfectant. I grabbed the scrotum and pulled it down to highlight the outline of the testes underneath. Next I made a quick light incision. One shiny white testicle popped out and hung there for a second. I heard a muffled voice say, 'Oh God!' and footsteps tripped away from me to the door a couple of yards behind me.

'Your friend doesn't look too good,' said Mr White. I had ignored this hiccup and removed the testicle. Then I quickly cut the other out.

'Leasden, are you okay?' I asked as I walked back to the door. I popped my head out of the byre. Leasden was leaning against the wall breathing heavily. He had crossed his legs and had his hands between his knees.

'Okay?' I asked with genuine concern

'Yes, I'm fine,' he responded, wiping his nose. 'It was a bit of a shock. They must be about the same size as human testes. It just caught me off my guard, that's all.'

'Fine, fine,' I said. 'They probably are – I have never thought of that before. Anyway, you just stay here. I'll just finish off this job.'

I moved back into the byre. Mr White stood against the wall with another calf for me to do. Soon we had finished. I checked the heads. They were no horn buds present.

'It seems to have worked.'

'Yes, that saves us doing another jobby,' agreed Mr White. 'You and your friend have time for a fly cup? He would be better of one. I think.' Leasden appeared quiet, almost sleepy.

'Good idea,' I said. 'Thank you.'

We all trooped into the kitchen. I saw Leasden look about himself in surprise. He was wide awake now. The kitchen was dilapidated. On our right as we came in stood a kitchen table hard against the wall with a window beside it. The panes were grimy such that only half the light entered. On the window sill were three small pots. One living cactus and two dead ones were inside. Opposite the kitchen table was a small coffee table pressed to a wall. Two ancient upholstered chairs sat on either side. Doors besides these chairs led to other rooms. On our left stood an Aga stove with a kettle on it and a teapot brewing tea. The stove was black. Above it a few clothes lines hung with great loops displaying threadbare clothes and cloths. Opposite the stove was a large sideboard overwhelmed with correspondence. Many of the envelopes were brown with stamps indicating official business. Hard by the sideboard was an old-style meat safe with metal grilles. The wallpaper for the room was a patterned pea-green colour that had a shade of brown-grey added to it due to the workings of the stove. A calendar donated by agricultural merchants was pinned against one wall.

On another wall hung a large oil painting. It was dark and it was difficult to discern the rural scene under the deposits layered on the painted surface. The skirting board round the edge was damaged in a peculiar way with little small spots, as though some fungus or rot had got at it. In a couple of places there were outright holes in the wood. Up above on the ceiling in two places small envelope-size pieces of paper were threatening to come down.

'Tea, Mother,' ordered Mr White, directing Leasden and myself to the table.

Mrs White, who was half bent with years of hard work, came forward. She placed three mugs on the table. She added the teapot from the stove. It looked as though it had come from a charity shop, as did a plate laden with biscuits. The biscuits by contrast were obviously home-made and edible. I stared at the mugs in surprise.

'What happened to the other mug?' I said. 'These here are brand new George VI Coronation mugs. Are you sure you want us to use them?' They seemed completely out of place.

'Well, that Jimmy finally broke that mug,' Mr White said, referring to his neighbour. 'Fine mug it was too. Edward VIII Coronation mug. So the handle was a bit deen. But he shouldn't ha' dropped it. Smashed. Smithereens. So we're now on to the next Coronation mugs. Also appropriate for your friend here.' He indicated Leasden.

I remembered the Edward VIII mug. All the visitors got it. It only had half a handle. Mr White himself used a big mug which simply said 'The Boss'. His wife used mugs sold by various charities.

We finished our tea and headed off, thanking them for the refreshment.

'Are you feeling okay?' I asked Leasden.

'Yes, I'm fine. Truly fine. I was caught by surprise. It won't happen again,' Leasden replied. 'Those people must be very poor. Such few possessions, and forced to use heirlooms such as Coronation mugs. I almost felt we should leave an offering – a fiver or something.'

'Now, there you are completely wrong!' I laughed. 'It's true the majority of farmers are not rich. However, Mr White and his brother are probably the richest people for miles around. He's worth a lot of money. He's just damn careful how he spends it.'

'I don't believe you!' said Leasden.

'Well, I know for a fact that during the early Nineties boom years one of the two once went to an independent financial advisor wanting to invest money. The advisor asked him what sum of money had he in mind. There and then he produced twenty thousand in cash hidden in a supermarket plastic bag. It was still damp. He had just dug it up.'

'Well I never!' said Leasden.

Our car approached a man walking down the road. He had a flat cap jammed down on his head. I recognised his gait. It was the neighbour, Jimmy, out checking his beasts. We slowed down. I wound down my window.

'Hello, Jimmy. How are you? Not bad weather, is it?' I asked.

'Nae bad, nae bad at a',' he replied, a big smile on his face. 'You been busyh vit? I s'ppose you've bin to Broomhill.'

'Aye, we did that,' I replied, 'amongst others.'

'Aye, he told me he had a puckle to cut. But said he wouldn't bother me.'

'He did that,' I agreed. 'We got new mugs to use.'

'Did you, by God!' smiled Jimmy. 'Did he tell you I brack the auld een? You should have speared at him exactly fit happened.'

'He practically told us,' I said.

'Aye, well there's another version. Right enough I dropped it. That's true. One morning last week he had me in for a fly cup, like. I wa' by the winner holding yon mug by the remains of the handle. Ye ken the middle wa missing you held it by twa wee bitties top and bottom?'

'Aye.' I was by now intrigued.

'Weel, I was jist aboot to tak a sip of tay. It was right by my lips when I heard a bloody great bang like a gun. Ma fist wobbled like this – ye ken?' Here he wobbled a bit. 'I tried to catch the mug but it got awa' from me – and doon it went and smithered itsell on the fleer. Some of the tay went o'er ma beets. So I turns to Angus to ask what the heel was that. Ye've nae idea fit I saw?'

'Na, na' I said.

'There is Angus sitting in his chair. Ye ken the een by the wee table. A bloody great gun in his lap smoking from one barrel.

'"*Jeeeesus!* For the love of God," I says. Because I now minded feeling a whoosh of air close to my back. But all Angus says is: "That's one bugger less." He points at the edge of the room behind me and there is these wee bitties of a moosey splattered all against the boarding and hole in it as weel.'

'Goodness!' I said.

'Well, I was at him. Fit why couldn't he git poison or a cat? Like ony reasonable buddy. But he turns on me and starts raging me for bracking his mug. I says I am lucky not to be a bloody moose. Onyway we calmed down a wee bit. Missus telt us all to had our tongues, and so that's it.'

'You're still speaking?' I asked.

'Of course we are,' he said. 'I'm not going to let a little thing like that ruin a good neighbour. Mind you, I'm buggered if I'm buying him a mug at the next coronation. I telt him that. He said it was fine by him.'

'Oh well, at least you're speaking,' I said. 'Well, nice to see you. We must go.'

'Aye, mustn't hinder you,' said Jimmy. 'Besides, I have a few beasts to check yet.'

We moved on.

'I thought the skirting board had dry rot and fungus,' commented Leasden. 'Now I see that it's defects have a more traumatic origin.'

'You could say that,' I agreed. 'But it's par for the course here.'

'He was quite broad, wasn't he?'

'He could be broader. In fact he was using a lot of English words just out of consideration to you and me. Mind you, I can catch most of them now. Better use the radio. Vet Three to base.'

'Hello, Richard. Mr Duncan is here with his box. I'll tell him you'll be here in ten minutes to quarter of an hour. Is that okay?' June replied.

'Fine that,' I said.

I parked the car at the back of the surgery and cleaned up. Then we went up to the front. June rose as I entered the office.

'Before you see the gentleman, Alec would like to have word with you.' She nodded toward a farmer standing at the window.

'Oh hello, Alec. How can I help?' I asked.

'I've got these calves indoors, like. They're all vaccinated and wormed but I think there's something working on them. They've been in a month or so.'

'They are still on their mothers?'

'Oh yes. They're only about three hundredweight. One or two a little scruffy, a touch of a cough. There are about fifty in the three buildings and I've treated three. I wonder if they are short of some minerals or something.'

'Do you feed a mineral?'

'Aye, there's something in the creep feed, but they may not all be taking it,'

'Well, we don't want to stress them by unnecessary handling. It's better if I came out, and we have it all set up to quietly take out about four or six. I can check them, perhaps take some temperatures and take some bloods for minerals and vitamins and the like... check the levels of Vitamin E in the creep feed and so on.'

'Aye, I think that would be fine. I think if I leave it, it could be trouble. I remember one year we had to do them all with vitamin E and selenium and the worst with tetracycline as well.'

'Could be the same again, but we'll see. Can you arrange a time with June for tomorrow? It's a bit too dark and late now.'

'Oh aye, aye fine, thanks.' Alec turned to arrange a time with June.

I went over to the man sitting with a styrofoam box beside him.

'Sorry to keep you,' I said, examining the record card June had given me. It was not filled in correctly. 'What have you got there? It is Mr Vine, isn't it?'

'Yes. I am. Actually I've got two matters I want to discuss with you,' he said, rising to his feet.

'Well, come in here.' I indicated the consulting room and closed the door with Alec's eyes following me.

'Yes,' I said. 'Fire away.'

'I keep one or two exotic animals as pets,' Mr Vine started. 'I worked on the rigs and then the oil company moved me all over the world. That's when I began this interest. I got advice and set up all the vivariums and aquariums with help from other enthusiasts.'

'Fine,' I said. It appeared that he was a competent keeper.

'Well, please don't laugh about what I'm going to ask you.'

'No, I won't.' Why did they always preface requests like this, I wondered. After all, I frequently stuck my hand in unimaginable parts of animals and that is taken seriously.

'I own a twelve-year-old piranha called Reg.' Mr Vine had gone a little pink.

'Is he in there?' I asked. I thought I might as well see him as hear about him.

'No, no, no,' said Mr Vine. 'I know he's ill. In fact, he must be pretty sick. Recently a large growth has formed on his side. I'm sure it's hopeless; that's why I didn't even bother bringing him here. I just want him put to sleep at home. It's okay – I am quite prepared to do it myself. I feel after all these years I owe it to him to do it quickly and painlessly. How do you do it?'

I came clean immediately.

'I don't know,' I shrugged my shoulders. 'The obvious answer is the priest. Just pick him out and hit him hard on the head. Once he's unconscious you can remove his head with impunity. It does occur to me to be a little rough as a method but it's efficient. Done all over the world that way.'

'Ya, I realise that.' Mr Vine sucked his breath in nervously. His eyes met mine in a beseeching manner. 'It's just that I wanted to do something. Oh, um, how do you say ... something with, I mean, something less obviously brutal. We've had him twelve years; I think that would be close to murder for me, battering him.'

'I tell you what,' I said, scratching my head. 'The chances are that what with whatever you have in that box I will be phoning a zoo or some other expert. When I do that I'll tell you their answer to your question. Is that fair enough?'

'Yes, yes, that's a good idea, thank you.' Mr Vine appeared genuinely relieved.

'Well, what is it?' My eyes flicked down to the box.

'Ah, this ...' said Mr Vine with excitement ... 'I keep snakes – quite a few – and I have started to breed them. Now this is an African rock python. She has laid three eggs but I think she's stuck with one more. I have all the other eggs incubating. I'll get her out for you. As you probably know she's a constrictor, but she has quite a nasty bite all the same.'

'Right,' I said. 'Can you get her out for us to examine?'

'Sure. Stand back a little. All doors closed?'

'Yes,' I said. Leasden and I stood back.

Expertly, Mr Vine took the snake from its cloth bag. I estimated it to be about nine feet long. It was light brown and there was a slight swelling about two-thirds down its length.

'It's quite cool here so that will slow her a bit,' said Mr Vine, holding it's head and a section near the tail. 'Do you want to feel?'

'Sure,' I said. She was cool and dry to touch, and I felt around the swelling and saw that this area was not too far from the cloaca.

'What we have to do,' I said, 'is to X-ray it to confirm the diagnosis. The egg should show up well. Then we'll have to take advice or I have to refer you to a snake reproductive man – a sort of snake gynaecologist. We'll just take it step by step. Is that alright by you?'

'Yes, great. Will you need a hand with the X-ray?'

'Yes, I think I would appreciate that. We won't hopefully need to knock her out, but I don't think many of my staff like handling these. Can you give me a minute or two to set it up? In the meantime you might put it back where it's warmer.'

I went next door and explained to June what we had to do. She confirmed that she wanted to avoid the snake. Leasden wandered in.

'I am bemused by the ethics of advising a client to batter his piranha,' he observed, po-faced. June froze.

'Are either of you on drugs or something?' she asked archly.

'No, June. It's only Leasden burbling,' I replied rapidly. 'We've got to concentrate on the matter in hand; the snake. We need to X-ray it.'

'*You* need to,' she stated abruptly.

'Right, right. Well, we need to do it before evening surgery. Any of the others around?'

'No!' June was not usually so unhelpful. It began to dawn on me that snakes were truly abhorrent to her

'Well, Leasden?' I asked.

'Yes, I'll help. Just tell me clearly what you need.'

'Right, follow me.'

We went to the X-ray room and set it up. Then we instructed Mr Vine what to do. I held the tail while he held the head. We stretched the snake briefly over the table. On my word once it had settled on the X-ray plate Leasden pressed the button. We put the snake away and took off our protective lead coats. June agreed to develop the X-ray. Five minutes later she returned. We gathered round the X-ray display box. It was obvious even to the untrained eye that there was an egg present in the snake.

Mr Vine and I discussed the matter briefly. I told him I would phone him as soon as I knew the possible courses of action. In the meantime he would go home and wait for my call late that afternoon. June was visibly relieved once the snake had left the premises.

I telephoned London Zoo. They put me through to a snake expert. He offered to do the job for three hundred pounds all in, but Mr Vine would have to get down there. He suggested I could have a go. He would give me directions for the anaesthetic. He explained the manipulation was fairly basic once the vet had familiarised himself with the anatomy. Before I rang off I suddenly remembered I had one more question.

'Excuse me asking, but I have another query; it is for real. Mr Vine also has an old piranha with tumours which he wants to euthanase. He doesn't want to use a priest and so on. Do you have any suggestions? Or is there a fish expert who could help me?' I kept my voice firm.

'Yes, we occasionally get asked that type of query. I know the answer. Is it in a fairly ordinary fish tank? Thirty inches by eighteen by eighteen?'

'I think so.'

'Well, so long as it isn't some big tank the size of three coffins the solution is simple. For an average tank he should put in three extra strength Alka-Seltzers. They alter the pH of the water rapidly and knock the fish out. Once that's done it'll belly up, out cold. He should get it then and apply the priest while it's unconscious. It may, however, not be necessary. The pills themselves may kill a sick fish.'

'Oh thank you, thank you very much! I'll pass that on. I'll get back to you about the snake.'

'Yes, and good luck. I think you'll be doing it.'

'I wonder,' I said as the phone went dead. I called Mr Vine and explained the possibilities about the snake. He said he would prefer we had a shot at it. So we agreed he would bring it in the next day at eleven a.m. once we had cleared away all the routine small animals.

'And did you remember about Reg?' asked Mr Vine.

'Yes, I did,' I said. 'The Zoo said put three or more Alka-Seltzers in the aquarium. It is a standard sized one, isn't it? Not something enormous, just a couple of feet or so?'

'Oh yes, it is quite an average size. We could never find any fish able to live for any length of time with Reg. So there was never a need for a big aquarium.'

'Quite.' What had they done? Undeterred, I carried on – 'I have never advised anyone of this before. Do you mind phoning back once you've done this? Purely out of professional interest, I would like to know if it works. Someone here can take a message for me.'

'Sure, I'll phone. Bye.' And he was gone.

I phoned London Zoo to say that I was on. The snake expert gave me some final advice. I took some detailed notes. Then we started the small animal surgery. Midway through it, Neil answered the phone, as everyone else was busy.

'Right,' I heard him say. 'Right, I'll pass on the message. I promise to pass it on, thanks. Yes, yes I will. Thank you for phoning.' He placed the phone down.

'Richard, I don't know who that was. In fact I don't pretend to want to know who phoned but he passed on a message for you. I got it down. "Reg floated belly up immediately. He has passed on without pain. Thank you, thank you." Make sense? I see you nodding: good, good. My, my, Richard, what a strange life you lead! June tells me you want to operate on a nine-foot African rock python tomorrow. Is this true?'

'Yes,' I said. 'I might need some help, if you're free.'

'No, you bloody well won't! I'm like June. That animal demonstrates my limit on exotics. Luckily I have a test of a hundred-odd cattle tomorrow. Sorry. I'll make sure you have help, but not me. Oh, and by the way, make sure the owner pays, won't you? Can't have you risking yourself for no reward.' Neil had stated his case.

'Don't worry, Neil. It'll be fine.' I put this forward as an article of faith. 'We just need to make sure we have time and space. I've cleared tomorrow's book for that time, except, of course, for your herd test.'

'Good.'

Chapter Twelve

We have scotched the snake, not killed it.

Macbeth, William Shakespeare

The next day we dealt with the morning surgery and then moved to the three small animals to operate on.

'Anne will do the male cat,' I said to Leasden. 'Meanwhile, I'll just spay this cat. Whoever finishes first will do the dog with the dental. Do you want to come and give me a hand? You've seen how Emma helped me before.'

'Sure,' replied Leasden.

I had this theory that for people who might be squeamish it's often better to get them to be busy. I directed him on how to put out the surgical instruments and prepare the cat. He shaved it and disinfected it well.

'That's fine, thank you,' I said. 'If you get yourself scrubbed up you can come and give me a hand.'

Soon Leasden and I were working through the operation. He was adept considering it was his first time at assisting a surgical procedure.

'That's great, thanks,' I said, as I finished stitching up the skin of the cat. 'If you just tidy it up. Emma will show you exactly how we can get ready for the next matter. Oh, and before I forget, my lady wife was asking if you would like to come for dinner soon. I will take your nod as a "yes".'

I left them to it and walked back to the office. A few minutes later Mr Vine appeared. He and I weighed the snake in its bag. Then I went back to the office and calculated the amount of ketamine that was needed. Next I filled a syringe with the required amount.

'We'll need to inject in a quiet warm place. I've set something up down the back. If you come with me and I'll get someone to help, then we'll give it the first anaesthetic.' I went next door for help. The girls were not enthusiastic.

'If it's unconscious, yes, I would love to help,' said June.

'Me too,' said Emma. 'Anne has just gone out for a second.'

I looked at Leasden.

'Me? Sure. Just tell me exactly what to do.'

Leasden, Mr Vine and I trooped down the back to an amateur vivarium I had made. We agreed to inject the snake and then pop it in. Mr Vine removed the snake and held it by the head and part of the hind coils. Leasden helped by holding more coils. Then we steadied her on a surface while I found a site to inject it.

'Ready?' I asked.

'Yes, ready,' they replied.

I lifted a scale and prepared to inject the snake through the skin. The zoo had directed me to avoid the scales as they were very difficult to repair. I pushed the needle in and felt the most incredible sensation come from the snake. It reacted with speed and tried to move its body. It was as though it was living steel. The strength and flexibility took me back completely. The syringe moved haphazardly in spite of my firm grip. In desperation I injected the ketamine.

'Right, pop her in!' I ordered. We quickly placed her in the vivarium and closed the lid. 'We'd better leave her now. The zoo said check her every few minutes or so. When she's out she'll be all limp. We won't have much time and will need to put her on gas anaesthetic pretty quickly.'

'That didn't go too bad,' commented Mr Vine.

'Incredible strength,' I said. 'I'd never realised it. It's no small wonder they can constrict.'

'Oh yes!' laughed Mr Vine as we left the room. 'You need to make sure someone else is around with her – in case the extra person has to unwind her from your neck!'

Five minutes later I went back to find the snake completely out. She had become unconscious much faster than the zoo had said. Fortunately, we had all the preparations to hand. I grabbed the limp python and rushed her up to the operating room. Once in there Emma opened its mouth to reveal a set of sharp teeth and the opening of the trachea well forward in the mouth just under the tongue. I slipped an endotracheal tube into the windpipe and we switched the gas on. The tube was designed for a cat, so June volunteered to place her hand at the tip of the snake to ensure the tube remained in place. Thus the snake received the anaesthetic and stayed unconscious. Emma and I moved further down the snake and, using stethoscopes, found the heartbeat. We also found the region of the snake where the lungs were placed. By watching this Emma could monitor the breathing and listen to the heart. She took out a piece of graph paper and began to note down these two parameters. The snake only breathed about once every forty seconds, but we had been warned it would be that slow. Mr Vine stood well back. Soon I had all that I wanted.

The snake was laid out on the length of the table with a few bends in it so as to fit on the table. At one end, June had the gas anaesthetic applied. A little further down on the same side of the operating table sat Emma, listening intently to the heart and the breathing and making records. There was an operating lamp behind me to give me good light and one or two pieces of equipment, including lubricating fluid and specula. I sat down and turned over the snake at the level of the cloaca. The egg was only about six inches short of the cloaca. I put some lubricating fluid into the cloaca. Then I looked up to the head of the table. I froze.

At the front June swayed a little and blinked. Then suddenly she vomited. A mass of semi-sold liquid went over the snake and the top of the table. I saw June's legs crumple, her eyes flutter and close. She keeled over and fell down by the table. I got up quickly and the operating light spun away from me and fell over. There was a loud *poof* as the light bulb inside imploded. Undeterred, I rushed toward June, knocking over a couple of drug bottles, which smashed on the floor. I got to June and noticed that she still had the anaesthetic tube in her hand. She had pulled it out from the snake. I bent down to check her and heard Emma behind me saying, 'The heart rate is going up and so is the breathing – I think it's waking up. We need more anaesthetic, June. June! Oh my God! June, what has happened to you? Oh my God, the snake! The snake's moving, June! The snake – it's moving, moving. June, June, June … oh, oh!'

Meanwhile I was clearing mess from June's mouth to establish an airway. I had no idea what had happened to her. Hearing Emma and seeing the useless anaesthetic tube in June's hand, I turned round and saw Mr Vine backing to the wall, his mouth opening and closing like a landed fish. Leasden, by contrast, was calm.

'Leasden!' I shouted. 'Grab the snake just behind the head and pin it to the table. With your other hand grab another part of it if you can. Emma, phone for an ambulance now. I have no idea what's wrong with June.'

I bent down to June again and lifted an eyelid. Her pupils were dilating and contracting. I had seen that with people that had fainted. She took a breath. There was no sound of any obstruction. I had already moved her legs into a first aid position. I bent down and listened and then in frustration grabbed a stethoscope. Again I listened; there was a strong regular beat. Emma came back.

'Here, let me look, Richard. I am a first-aider, remember. The ambulance is coming.'

'Okay,' I said. 'I'll sort this snake out.' We changed positions.

I grabbed the anaesthetic tube and turned round to Leasden. The snake was writhing slowly but was not moving, thanks to Leasden's firm grip.

'We'll just try and pop this back in,' I told him. With that I prised open the mouth. The snake's jaw champed at me but I had used a blunt instrument to get a view of the mouth. I saw the tongue and the hole just below it where the windpipe started. I pushed the tube in and the eyes opened in shock for a split second. It swallowed.

'Right, Leasden, you and I will just have to stay like this until it calms down and goes out again. I can't turn up the anaesthetic – we might lose it if it goes too deep suddenly. I don't fancy ventilating a comatose snake.'

I heard noises behind me. June was coming to. Outside there was the sound of hurried steps.

'In here!' shouted Emma.

A fully equipped paramedic, resplendent in green boiler suit, stepped in. His professional eyes immediately fixed on the semi-supine body of June.

'June! I wondered if it was you,' he said as he took a pace forward.

'Hi, Garry! I'm okay, honest – just a turn, that's all.'

Garry then glanced around. His eyes took in the vomit on the table, the smashed medicine bottles, the fallen operating lamp, and the snake moving slowly.

'For the love of God, what have you guys been up to?'

'Only operating on a snake in labour,' I replied quietly.

'Well, whatever,' he said brusquely. 'I'm taking June out now. Me and my colleague will check her over and then we'll probably take her home to relax for the rest of the day. Dean – don't look in here, it's a mess. Just get the chair ready and we'll take June out now. Come here, June; never mind the mess.' He bent down and lifted June up and took her out.

'I'm okay, really,' said June. 'Seriously, just a turn.' They left the room.

'Easy, Dean,' we heard from next door. 'There! You're chaired, June. Now we're taking you away from those odd folk you work with all day.'

We all looked at each other.

'Oh, well,' smiled Emma, shrugging her shoulders. 'Better get on. I'll just tidy this up if you want to carry on.'

We could all see the snake was moving less and less.

'Good idea,' I said. 'Leasden, you keep that anaesthetic tube in and keep an eye out for the breathing while Emma tidies up. It breathes about once very forty seconds or so. You keep an eye on the clock on the wall for that. Are you sure June will be okay, Emma? What do you think?'

'June'll be okay, Mr Jones, I'm sure of that,' she said with a surreptitious smile. 'She quite likes that Garry. He's a hunk, if you know what I mean.'

I shrugged my shoulders and returned to the last third of the snake. Once again I started manipulating the egg and squeezing it gently down to the cloaca. Bit by bit it moved until we could begin to see it. At this juncture it would have been easier for me if I had punctured the egg. Once it collapsed it would come out easily. But I knew Mr Vine wanted a whole egg. Eventually, with one final squeeze, it came out. Mr Vine suddenly became mobile and bounced forward to collect the egg. He had a little nest to hand for it. He retired to the back clutching his precious cargo. We then decided to let the snake come round. With remarkably little ceremony, Mr Vine departed. He needed to rush back and place mother and egg in safe warm quarters. He stuffed the relevant cash in my hand.

'Well, that's that. What an event!' The operating theatre still showed one or two signs of recent drama. 'Emma, can you phone June at home and check she's okay? She'd be better taking the rest of the day off. I'll phone the Zoo to check if there's any more follow-up needed.'

A few minutes later Emma reported back. June was fine. She apologised but she hadn't had much breakfast and what with that and the other matters had fainted. I hinted there was no need for her to apologise. I went off to phone the Zoo.

'How did you get on?' asked the expert.

'Oh, success, I think,' I said, but I omitted to describe the operation in full detail. I wondered if there was any follow-up needed.

'No, it should be okay,' said the expert. 'Unfortunately, the egg is almost certainly infertile. In fact, if you give me his phone number I'll have a chat with Mr Vine. I don't usually do this, but I think in the circumstances I will to avoid him blaming you if there's any disappointment. As long as the snake has an appetite she'll be okay. He just has to try again and get another clutch of eggs. Anyway, well done. You've saved her, which is the main thing.'

I gave him my thanks. That was probably the end of the business. We had to return to more local matters.

'Can Anne cover for me if I go to lunch now?' asked Emma. 'June isn't here to cover, and Anne has just got back.' I nodded agreement. 'Also, I think you should take an early lunch and then head off to Mrs Gall in the Glacks early afternoon.'

'Fine,' I said. 'Leasden, we can meet back at or soon after one p.m.'

At one o'clock Leasden and I headed back to the Glacks. The radio suddenly came alive.

'Base to Vet Three.' It was Neil.

'Yes, I'm here,' I said.

'Richard, what have you done to June?' Neil sounded excited.

'She just fainted, that's all,' I replied.

'I can see in spite of the tidy-up one or two things were broken. He did pay, didn't he? Not to put too fine a point on it, we have to break even, you know. Senior partners, old complaint.'

'Yes, Neil, he paid up in cash,' I said to soothe him.

'That's something, and I gather the snake is going to live?'

'Yes.'

'Good. I'm glad you handled it. Over.'

Ten minutes later Leasden and I were back at Mrs Gall's. She was waiting for us. We went in to see Brig. We bent low to get in the building. He looked much brighter. Mrs Gall was relieved. We took off the styrofoam soles. They had been crushed from an inch and a half to a little longer than half an inch. I pared these compressed pieces because they had to be replaced in addition to an extra sole for Brig to compress again. Leasden held the head while Mrs Gall and I slowly went round from foot to foot.

'I'm so glad this seems to be working,' she said.

'Aye, it makes it worthwhile all this work,' I agreed.

'It's not just that,' went on Mrs Gall, 'but to us this is something that effects us all in the house. It's like a member of the family being sick.'

'Yes, it is tricky, isn't it?'

'Of course, you see this all the time, and you're most likely thinking about technical matters. So it doesn't quite come home to you,' she suggested.

'Yes and no,' I explained. 'We often do feel for you but we can't let it affect us; otherwise we'd go nutty. So, yes we do set up some sort of barrier – if only to do the job right and think clearly and objectively.'

'And all the while you have wailing females around you ruining your train of thought!' she laughed.

'Yes, yes, I suppose so,' I said. 'I have had that. Funnily enough Neil comes in for it more than me. He just puts his head down and does the job. He's gentle in what he does, it's just on occasion he has a cool manner some don't understand. They don't realise he's concentrating on the animal's needs. Some people think he doesn't care. That is certainly not true. I've known him to come back, and once he's sitting down to be quite upset, particularly if he has seen an animal in some pain. But at the time he's with the animal he disciplines himself to be cool.'

'I could see how that could be mistaken,' said Mrs Gall quietly.

'The interesting thing is that over time people who meet us realise that we vets really *do* care, even the vets who don't show much emotion … One more foot and we're done.'

A couple of minutes later we all stood up. As if on cue one of the daughters appeared. She went straight to the head of Brig and almost snatched the head collar from Leasden. She started talking to the horse.

'See what I mean?' smiled Mrs Gall. 'Teenagers may have no manners but by golly they have emotions. Oh, by the way, Anne phoned me and I've arranged to pick up some feeds from the surgery tomorrow.'

'Fine, we'll be on our way,' I said. 'I'll phone to arrange a visit to take those shoes off. Have you got a farrier coming?'

'Yes, tomorrow,' she replied. 'At last I pinned one down and he'll come down. He said something about dumping the toes.'

'Yes, he'll do one or two things like that to reduce the chances of the bone rotating. Hopefully the risk is small now; anyway, if he needs to speak to me ask him to phone. He will most likely manage himself.'

We departed.

'Vet Three to base,' I radioed in.

'Can you go to Noyes at Garroughburn, please, Richard?' Emma replied. 'He has a calf not thriving. He's there now.'

'Right,' I answered. Then I turned to Leasden. 'We'll have to walk the last part. He's over the burn.'

I drove further up the Glack and then turned down to the burn. Five yards short of it I stopped. The track went down to the burn, but I knew it was too deep for the Laguna, and the bottom of the burn was very uneven at that point. We took some drugs in a box. I guided Leasden to a point a few yards downstream. Here there were large stones crossing the water. We didn't need to leap from stone to stone but only had to walk to the right of them. At that spot, although the water flowed by at speed, the burn was shallow. There were hidden slabs on the river bed. Leasden got up on the bank first and faced me, with clumps of reed either side of him. I passed him the box and then heaved myself out. We looked up. About two hundred yards up the hill stood the farm buildings. Smoke came out slowly from a crooked chimney. We walked up the stone-strewn track with a measured tread and saved our breath for the walking. When we were ten yards short of the nearest low building, out popped Mr Noyes. He was a short, slightly stooped old man with great long bushy white eyebrows that would have been the envy of any owl. He sucked on a pipe but it was not alight. The doctor had ordered that a few years ago.

'Ach, vit,' he said. 'It's been a long time. And I see you have yer fether fer company.'

'He's a teacher-cum-student,' I tried to explain the unexplainable.

'Fitever.' Mr Noyes dipped his head and disappeared into a low farm building typical of any old croft. We followed. It was dark. I stood. There was no point in advancing into the unknown. At length my eyes became accustomed to the twilight conditions. Mr Noyes stood with all the time in the world.

'There he is,' he stated. 'I jist git him here for handiness.'

I could see the calf. He was only about two hundredweight. He appeared very scruffy and his forehead dipped inwards in manner characteristic of a poor-thriving beast.

'Has the mother any milk?' I asked.

'Ony milk!' he spurned my suggestion that the calf was undernourished. 'She's a demn good milker. I even tak a sip mysel'. But I dinna tak such that I rob the calf. Na, something else is ado.'

'Well, we'd better get a had of him.' I moved forward, as did Mr Noyes. One advantage of the dull light was that the calf was a little slow at moving. He tried to move away but Mr Noyes held him; although the farmer was short and wiry this belied his true strength. Once I had seen him effortlessly lift the tow bar of a heavy trailer. It was a feat I could not imitate. I examined the calf; I could feel his heart pounding away and he seemed a little breathless.

'Leasden, could you bring the box? Is there a torch there?'

Leasden looked in and replied in the negative.

'I've a lighter,' offered Mr Noyes.

'Fine that,' I said. 'Jist light it here at the shoulder blades. Mind not to burn the calfie.'

'I'll be careful,' he said. His lighter gave a flame as I parted the hairs. It was black near the skin.

'I think this calf is covered in lice.'

'Na,surely no?' said Mr Noyes.

'Here, look,' I demonstrated, holding some hairs I had plucked with lice attached. We peered at the specimen. Eventually Mr Noyes caught sight of them.

'Bey Christ, it's full of yon beasties!' he said.

Leasden afterwards said it had been like viewing a painting by Caravaggio. The shadows cast by the single light had been thrown all around the room, while over the vet and farmer's faces the flame had highlighted the shadows or reflections of creases, eyebrows, lips, stubble and so on. The sudden expression of disbelief by Mr Noyes had been memorable.

'Move the light down to the mouth,' I requested him. This he did. I revealed the gums by moving the lips. The gums were very pale. 'He's very pale. The lice are taking a fair sip of his blood. This would account for nearly all the problems. Can you hold on to him? I'll get some injections from the box. Then you'll have to come to the surgery for some pour-on for all the calves. In fact, I would do the cows as well. This infestation is pretty heavy. Are there any others similar?'

'Na, na,' Mr Noyes answered. 'One or two flecking a bit but none as bad as this.'

'All the same, I do recommend you do them all,' I said. 'Else you may be calling me back to treat another.'

'Richt, richt, I'll dee them a',' he said hastily. 'I'll come doon for the pour-on or fitever tomarra.'

I injected the calf. 'He should be okay, Mr Noyes. One of the drugs I gave just now kills all lice that suck blood. Still, I would give him pour-on as well when you get it.'

We left Mr Noyes standing all alone by the farm building. Leasden and I made our way down the steep track to the burn.

'How common is it to find lice these days?' asked Leasden.

'It's uncommon to find a heavy infestation like that, I grant you,' I explained. 'However, the lice are always around. That's their job – to parasitise – and they are good at it. Why, even sheep scab, one of the simplest to get rid of, is making a comeback. It is a combination in that case of human incompetence and an efficient parasite.'

'Still, he had quite a few on that calf, didn't he?' pressed Leasden.

'Oh, I see, you are suggesting that he's a bad farmer? Well, it's funny you say that, and some textbooks would agree with you. But there's another way to look at it. If a heavy infestation of lice is his only major problem then he's not a bad farmer. Here, let me give you a hand.' I helped Leasden lower himself into the burn.

'How do you mean?' he asked.

'Well, he has none of those problems that we saw, for instance, of low vitamin E levels in fast-growing calves on special diets. He has no calf pneumonia problems, neither does he need tricky vaccination schedules against calf respiratory disease. He hardly buys anything in, and when he does he isolates the animal for a fortnight in one of those byres. I remember someone once showing me a slide of Moroccan farms dotted across high mountains. All the beasts in those farms were healthy and well isolated.'

'How peculiar!' said Leasden in surprise.

'Yes, there's always another way to see these things. I'm not an out-and-out advocate for completely *au naturel* farming, if you see what I mean. But provided you don't set your production targets too high and are prepared to live the lifestyle of Mr Noyes, you can farm well and—' I paused as Leasden pulled me out of the water at the far side of the burn— 'leave the land in a better state than when you got it. Soil is important stuff. That thin mantle of brown stuff we call earth – along with water, oxygen, CO_2, and light – is what keeps us alive. Sorry, I'm preaching, but soil is important and I'm a little fed up with people who cast unthought out criticism at Mr Noyes and those of his ilk.'

'I think I've touched a raw nerve,' hinted Leasden.

'Perhaps you have. I'm sorry,' I apologised. 'Let me put it this way: farmers have received as bad a press as politicians recently. Unfortunately, farmers themselves are not very good at presenting their case well. Too often it's the big boy farmers of large estates or the grieves of big farms who stand up to represent farmers. But these men don't stand for Mr Noyes. It's sad.'

We got back into the car. I radioed in.

'Vet Three to base,' I said.

'Richard, could you go to Terry at Crossfolds?' asked Emma. 'He's had a four-month calf die suddenly. It's probably not an anthrax investigation at so young an age – what do you think?'

'Well, I will make a judgement when I see it. Mind you, with the time of day you may find it difficult to get someone in at the Ministry. Anyway, we'll see. He wants a post-mortem?'

'Yes, that's the picture,' agreed Emma.

A quarter of an hour later we arrived at the farm. We met Terry and walked round the back. Lying on a trailer was a calf. It looked as though someone had tried to blow it up so as to mimic the Michelin man. The thighs were round and twice their normal size. It was obvious gas was underneath the skin.

'When did this die? I asked. 'It's terribly blown up. This could be gas gangrene or blackleg when blown up like this. Mind you, the weather's a bit too cold for it.'

'Oh, it hasn't been long dead,' replied Terry. 'At least, it was alive this morning. Died quite quickly.'

'Has there ever been blackleg here on this farm?'

'No, never. This is a home-bred beast. They're on a special mix as an extra feed. I blame that for causing bloat and killing it. Mind you, there is bicarbonate in it to reduce the risk.'

'The bicarbonate will be mainly for excess barley and acidosis, not bloat by itself. But anyway, we'd better see. I have these knives to hand.' I stuck a knife in the thigh and gas ripped out.

'Amazing!' I said. 'Well, gas has to be part of this story. It's a fresh carcase.' I nicked the abdomen, which was as tight as a drum. Gas came out under pressure and the animal hardly changed shape. The pressure was very great. A little foam appeared.

'That's odd,' I said. 'That is like frothy bloat when you feed cattle well-ground barley and little else.'

'There's a lot of roughage in the diet,' replied Terry.

'Well, years ago when I saw barley beef doing this we used to open their sides to save them from dying of bloat,' I went on. 'We had to make a big hole because the foam would not go through any trocar or pipe of small dimension. There was always a dramatic woosh of yellow stuff with the consistency of fire extinguisher foam. Let's see.' I made a bigger nick in the exposed rumen. Green-yellow foam shot out. It continued to spurt out well beyond the side of the trailer.

'By gum, that's it!' I said quite excited. 'Look, Terry, this is just pure foam.' I put some on my glove and it had a fascinating consistency: part mousse, part blancmange and part foam. To my surprise there was also a lot of fibrous matter.

'You see, the animal can belch up free gas,' I explained, 'but this foam it is unable to belch up and so the poor beast blows up in a few hours and dies.' Terry, I could see, was less excited. 'Anyway,' I continued, 'I'll look at one or two other body organs. Let's just try and look at the lungs.' I cut down to the site where the lungs are normally found and instead discovered foam-filled intestine.

'When it blows up it compresses the lungs then as well?' asked Terry.

These farmers are quick, I thought. 'Yes,' I responded. 'That must be why I'm finding gut pushed far up here. The diaphragm has been moved forward by all that pressure. Here, I've found a piece of lung. They all look normal. So does the heart. The liver's a little pale and so are some of the muscles.'

'But that foam would be the main cause?' asked Terry.

'Yes, definitely. But it's odd usually for froth like this to be found in an indoor four-month beef calf. It's more often found in cattle on pasture particularly with lots of clover. Or it's indoors on a ration with little roughage and well-ground barley.'

'Well, Richard, you can see the roughage in the foam. They get a lot of silage as well. The mix has pellets in it.' Terry showed me the mix of green pellets, brown pellets and barley. 'I can contact the feed people and see what can be done. In the meantime I'll take them off this feed and give silage only.'

'Right,' I agreed. 'I'll have to do some homework, because it's a little odd. In the meantime I'll give you some surfactants to treat any others you see in the next few hours. Any bad ones, call us out and if necessary stick the animal yourself on the left side. Also, I do remember the foam is not stable to movement: sometimes a little jog around a farm building destabilises the foam and settles the mildly affected ones. I'll phone you later this evening.'

We had a quick walk around the beasts. There were no others to see affected. As we left Terry was removing the suspect feed from some troughs.

'More complicated than Mr Noyes,' I murmured to Leasden.

'Does that mean you disapprove of the way he's farming?' asked Leasden.

'Not at all,' I said in an amused tone. 'I think both are equally valid.'

'Then what are your criteria for validity?' Leasden homed in on me.

'Well, it's none of your business,' I said a little irritated.

'No, Richard,' pursued Leasden. 'I would like to know. You are, after all, involved in this industry.'

'That's precisely it!' I fumed. 'I don't regard farming primarily as an industry. It is an industry; that is correct. But it is primarily a source of good wholesome food for a nation. It's a building block for life. Just like water is needed for living. Our island history tells us that we must treasure this building block of life. Remember, history tells us we nearly starved in the Second World War.'

'I am sorry to jump on another raw nerve,' Leasden was still calm. 'But I come again to your criteria for validity. If it's not a national industry, what is it?'

'My criteria is support for family farmers,' I said this with some tension. 'These families live on the farm for generations. They're not landlords or commercial firms who employ labourers and managers. Many landlords command from a great distance away from the farm. Sure, some family farmers are efficient, others not so; but they care for the land more than an industry. They and their children have to live on it. That is a security for a nation. If it's wholesome enough for them to live on and eat the produce it stands a better chance overall of being good for others. Of course, you'll be able to cite me the odd farm that destabilises this view. But one last point: the standard of animal well-being is often better on these family farms. It's different from welfare. Sorry, I've gone on … Vet Three to base.'

'Nothing new except a little job back here,' responded Emma.

'What might that be?'

'While the others do most of the small animals could you scan a few sheep for us?' Emma's voice had a suggestion of pleading. 'I'll set it up down the back. Harold has some gimmers he thinks might be empty. They should be lambing in a month.'

'Oh,' I sighed. 'Righto. It's an odd time to scan but let's give it a go. Put the head thing on which we got from the medics, please.'

As soon as we arrived back I cleaned my kit and was about to pack it away when Harold turned up. The first thing we saw was the back end of a trailer slowly nosing its way into the rear car park.

Harold brought in the gimmers – young ewes – one by one. Inside Emma had set up the scanner on a table. By one foot of the table was a small bucket of water with the scanner head. I lubricated the groin area of a gimmer while Harold held it sitting on its rear with its back straight. This was a similar position to that used for shearing sheep. Then I pressed the round scanner head into the groin. Harold had told me they should be well on in lamb. The young tup lamb had 'keeled' them all, but he was not sure they were in fact settled. We were looking for dark holes in the screen display. These would indicate fluid-filled sacs with hopefully embryos inside them. The first six showed no signs of pregnancy. This began to confirm his worst fears. The only fluid-filled sac we could find was almost certainly the bladder. The rest of the display screen just displayed gritty matter; if we left the probe in place we could see these moving slowly like slugs. They were just intestines.

'Have you got one you're sure is pregnant?' I asked.

'Yes, I have one. She was done by another tup. I'll get her now,' replied Harold.

'I think you should do that,' I concurred. 'We don't usually scan at over four months of pregnancy, so if you can get one for me we can double-check what it looks like. Mind you, it should be obvious with cotelydons from the placenta sticking out, and even a bone or two of the embryo.'

Harold brought in the known pregnant animal. I placed the probe on.

'I can see that's pregnant,' said Harold looking at the screen. 'It's completely different to see.' Sure enough, we could see vast spaces of darkness due to foetal fluids, and little bumps going into the fluid were the cotelydons where. Then we found a lamb.

'Bugger, what a mess!' expostulated Harold. 'Nearly all those thirty gimmers must be empty. I'll have to go away and think about this.'

'Well, you still have time,' I said. 'This part of the flock will have to change from early lambers in January to late lambers. It's still possible.'

'Aye, aye, I can do that,' agreed Harold. 'But I'm so annoyed with myself. I advise on tups to everybody and often tell them to make sure they have enough around to do the job right. And look what I've done with my own bloody gimmers, just left them with a tup lamb and no double-check! When he keeled them I assumed no problem. Been too busy elsewhere.'

'Sorry about that.'

'Ach, it's not your own fault. Anyway, thanks – at least I know exactly what is happening or not happening now.'

Leasden and I tidied up and then went forward to the office.

'You have quite a few phone calls to make, Richard,' Emma informed me. 'Two of your last Caesars want times to arrange to remove stitches. The cows are fine. You need to phone Terry about that feed. It's all in the book.'

I read the daybook. Sure enough, there were a number of calls to be made.

I finished the day phoning and making plans for tomorrow. In discussion with Terry he said he had checked the silage to find it had been full of clover, the barley had been fine ground and we had suspicion that some of the grass pellets might have had some high protein herbage in them or alfalfa. One of the three could be causing the problem or a little from all three. The best course was to use the feed in some other way but take those stock off it today.

As I left I reminded Leasden that my wife expected him to dinner the next day.

Chapter Thirteen

Dixeris egregie notum si callida verbum
Reddiderit iunctura novum.

You may gain the finest effects in language by the skilful
setting which makes a well known word new.

Horace, 65–8 BC

The next evening I was at the top of the house in my room. An
American would have called it 'the Den'. This was the only room
Jill had not ruled on for the exact form of the decorations. I was
tidying up my collection of cartoon books. The recently acquired
Giles cartoon books had been placed near another of the greats:
Pont.

A *stomp, stomp, stomp* noise heralded the arrival of teenage
offspring. Sure enough, Edward's head came round the door.

'There's a Mr Leasden downstairs to see you, Dad,' he said,
somewhat truculently.

Why, I wondered, is everything to do with parents a pain to a
teenager? 'Thanks, Edward.' I bottled my venom. 'Could you
guide him up here, please?' The suggestion was greeted with a
great sigh.

Three minutes later *stomp, stomp, stomp* accompanied by *step,
step, step* approached. Leasden and Edward entered.

'There, Father,' said the truculent one. Then, to show he was
not all bad, he carried on. 'Father, may I take the liberty to
introduce you to Mr Claude Leasden. Mr Jones: Mr Leasden. Mr
Leasden: Mr Jones.' With that he fled quickly down the stairs,
bang, bang, bang.

There was an embarrassing pause. It was filled with the sound
of Bruch's violin concerto.

'Ah, that is Bruch,' Leasden identified the piece. 'It's good music.'

'Yes, yes, it is. I put it on for background while I order my cartoon collection.'

'*Background?*' Leasden appeared stunned. 'Bruch never intended it to be background. This is great music. That is almost barbarism.'

For the second time that night I bottled my venom. In my own house, could I not play whatever I wanted to play? If I wanted to dance a jig to Mahler or Sibelius or listen intently for hidden depths in 'Who killed Cock Robin?' was that not my privilege?

'Perhaps you have a point,' I said mildly. 'These great romantics deserve respect. You're a bit of a romantic yourself, are you not?'

Leasden was a little ruffled. Days later I recollected I should have made a definite note of this uncharacteristic reaction of his. He changed the subject.

'These butterflies on the walls, are they yours?' Leasden was examining the room. The ceiling bent in at the edges parallel to the roof just above. All the paintwork was plain white. It was covered here and there by my bric-a-brac: display cases of butterflies; framed photographs; and a map of the world with pins in it. Trinkets from abroad could be found on top of the four bookshelves tucked low round the walls. A small bow window kept a round oak table in its centre. The table was covered with papers and had two captain's chairs set beside it.

'Oh yes, they're from all over the tropics, wherever my dad or I went. The main bulk is in the Boothe Museum. Those on the wall are just a few display boxes.'

'A few display boxes!' For once he seemed genuinely impressed. 'They are magnificent! Where did these come from?' he asked, pointing to one box.

'Those are West African. I used to walk through a lot of jungle to catch those.'

'Did you not find it dangerous?'

'Not really. You just have to be careful and keep your ears open. The only animal I ever came close to was a tapir, in Central America. Everyone's frightened of man in the jungle, and so was I. The most dangerous thing to meet in the jungle may well be another man.'

'Really?'

'Oh, yes! In Central America if you met a man he might be guarding a marijuana patch. He might shoot before he asked any questions. Plenty of room in the jungle for a shallow grave. That aspect is creepy.'

'So what did you do?'

'If I could, I would avoid any others in the jungle. Give them a wide berth or be still. As I said, you just keep quiet and use your eyes and ears.'

'And these butterflies are a fraction: the rest are in the museum? I mean, the main collection.'

'Yes, that's one of my few claims to well: not fame, but difference. Once the museum titled me "a bona fide collector"; I was proud of that. I wasn't out collecting for my own benefit but for scientific reasons. The numbers of insects in those jungles is incredible. I was very lucky. Given the chance I would love to go back. But to many it would seem very dull. Really, it's a lot of trees and darkness. It's an acquired taste, and some would prefer what you do – hill walking; I can understand that.'

'I think I wouldn't like the insects biting me,' Leasden observed.

'Well, you have a point there,' I laughed. 'They used to eat me a bit. Xavier, my Mayan assistant, used to say that they could smell fresh new blood and went for that. Hence they used to bite me more than him.'

'I see you also take a large number of photographs,' observed Leasden. 'You did that at college, did you not?'

'Yes, and I've carried on. It's a fairly typical hobby for a vet. But if you had time to examine what vets get up to in their spare time you would find my activities are by comparison fairly plain. There are many who parachute, scuba-dive, mountaineer and so on. As a professional bunch we seem to like – I think the expression is "pushing the envelope".'

'It's something like that. Mind you, my niece is training to get a pilot's licence.'

'There you go, Leasden. She's a classic example of what many vets get up to. My walking the jungle is small beer.' I winked at him.

Stomp, stomp, stomp.

'Mum says supper's ready. Can you come down now, please?' Edward announced.

'Yes, fine,' I said and we all filed down the steps. The kitchen table was laid.

'I thought we could eat in the kitchen. It's informal but more homely,' Jill gushed at Leasden.

'Oh, thank you,' said Leasden, and sat down. The children also sat down; their lips were motionless but their eyes moved communicating knowing glances that only they understood.

'It's venison tonight,' announced Jill. 'I gather you may have had a hand in this?'

'Well, no,' advised Leasden. 'I was only an observer. If anyone literally had a hand in it, it was Anne.'

'Gross!' commented Rachel.

'Do either of you want to be vets?' asked Leasden.

'Na,' replied Edward.

'No, no way,' added Rachel.

'Lawyer, either of you?' continued Leasden

'Na.'

'No.'

'You see what we have to put up with, Mr Leasden?' explained Jill. 'Still, they have plenty of time to consider what to do with their lives. You do like venison, I hope?'

'Oh yes, delicious, thank you,' responded Leasden.

'Dad said you would eat anything,' noted Edward.

'Edward!' I said, attempting to halt this line of thought.

'It's okay – let him go on.' Leasden was unabashed. 'I've probably heard worse.'

'Dad said you were fit enough to have a schoolboy for breakfast. Also that you were so harsh you'd swallow anything. Almost as though you were a cannibal.' Edward was unstoppable.

'Have you heard worse than that, Mr Leasden?' asked Rachel.

'Oh yes,' he retorted blithely. 'Mind you, your dad didn't like Classics. That might have something to do with it, don't you think?'

'Was there a subject you couldn't stand, Mr Leasden?' asked Edward.

'Oh yes – physics,' he satisfied their curiosity. 'I hated physics with a terrible passion.'

'Cool,' said Edward. 'Did you hate your physics teacher then?'

'Oh yes, with a malicious hatred.'

'Oh, magic!' enthused Rachel. 'What did you want to do to him?'

'Blow him up,' said Leasden, as though he was describing purchasing fish and chips. 'Unfortunately, I was so bad at physics that I didn't have the correct knowledge to make a decent explosive device.'

'Dad, your Classics teacher is one cool dude!'

'Yes, Mr Leasden, you must come more often,' said Rachel.

'Well, I am worried that these children don't read enough,' said Jill, attempting to steer the conversation in new directions. She handed round the vegetables.

'You mean all that they have read with care and understanding is the instruction manual to a PlayStation 2?' asked Leasden. 'Is that not true?'

'This man is *hot*,' said Rachel.

'Yes, he seems to understand us teenagers,' added Edward. He turned to stare at his mother. 'Unlike our geek-like parents.'

'A little rude that comment, I think, Edward,' chided Leasden.

'Well, anyway, perhaps you're correct,' Jill went on. Teenage insults disturbed her little. 'Maybe it's only the manuals that they read. You see they know almost nothing of literature. If it wasn't for JK Rowling and her books, I doubt they would've happily read any book themselves.'

'The PlayStations and the computers are a great and real attraction,' remarked Leasden. 'I never had them, and possibly you may also have just missed them.'

Jill coloured at the compliment to her youth.

'Well, I don't know. All I wish is that they read something good, like Shakespeare or Chaucer.'

'Not Chaucer,' said Leasden suddenly. Rachel's left eyebrow shot up. Edward's ears pricked. 'I mean, it's a little too mature. The style of English is difficult to understand. Even when translated it is a little antiquated and boring.'

'Oh, really?' said Jill noncommittally,

'Yes,' Leasden hurried on. 'I would opt for Swift – *Gulliver's Travels*. Or Dickens, or Austen.'

'Well you're the expert,' Jill allowed.

'Even Solzhenitsyn, wouldn't you say, Richard?'

'Yes, Solzhenitsyn.' I decided to help out. 'I would try him. It can be gripping – *The First Circle*, *Cancer Ward* and all that.'

'Are these all fiction?' asked Edward.

'Yes, they all are,' Leasden agreed. 'Why, don't you like that? Do you prefer fables or old stories with meaning?'

'No. I don't know,' Edward searched for words. 'I prefer history – facts and so on. But unfortunately it's often boring.'

'Truth is often stranger than fiction, Edward,' said Leasden, tutoring.

'Really? I'm not so sure.'

'Well, after this meal,' said Leasden, 'we could possibly demonstrate that. Let us see if we can get a true story from your parents. For instance, how they met and fell in love and so on. I will tell a fable, a modern fable. You can judge which is more interesting. Real life is full of surprises, you know.'

'Good,' said Rachel. 'I've never heard that story in full, about Mum and Dad. It may be embarrassing, but so what?'

I glanced at Jill. She winked.

'Fine by me,' she said. 'Then we're agreed: Mr Leasden's fable against our grand old romance, as told by Dad.'

'Hardly a great romance,' I said hurriedly. I found some red wine to settle my stomach and passed it round. The children opted for Irnbru.

Three-quarters of an hour later we were all gathered next door in the living room. Uncharacteristically, the children had remained. Normally they would depart to computers and PlayStations. This time they were both intent in hearing more.

'Right,' said Jill. 'What shall we have first? Truth or fable?'

'*Truth*,' was the unanimous vote. I cleared my throat.

'It was a dark and stormy night…'

The effect was explosive.

'My dad's first line, how embarrassing!' exclaimed Rachel. 'I think I'm going to be sick – and it's not Mum's cooking!'

'You have to admit, Father,' Edward followed up, 'that is a very poor opening line. Certainly lacks originality.'

'But,' I said, 'January the fourth 1982 *was* a dark and stormy night.'

'I think your father,' Leasden came in as an arbiter, 'is trying to explain that his opening statement is factually correct. Believe it or not, there was no attempt at literary excellence or literary absurdity. He just stated the plain fact without thinking.'

'See! See! He remembers the exact date.' Jill was perched neatly on top of a small Chinese lacquer stool. A big smug smile ran all over her face. She looked like a bumblebee high on nectar. She waved her fingers in command. 'On you go, on you go, Richard. Never mind the bairns...'

'To please the other members of the audience,' I continued, 'the weather was very bad. That night the TV had weather warnings on. A young man was waiting by the phone. He was a recent graduate from Cambridge up in the far north of Scotland on duty for the night. I remember hoping the phone would not go: all I had for company was a small cat in a small cold bungalow. But then the phone *did* ring and the senior partner asked me to go out to a calving.'

'"Have you done many calvings?" he had asked me.

'"Two," I said, "and both of them the calf was dead before I started."

'"Well, Mr Black only calls us out if there's a problem," confided the senior partner. "Still, do your best. Now he doesn't think you can manage all the way up to the farm. Have you a map there?"

'"Yes," I replied.

'"Can you see Gullyknowes?"

'"Yes."

'"There is a fork just north of it. He'll meet you there."

'"I can see it. Right, I'll go now."

'"Good, I'll listen out for you on the radio. If you get stuck, tell me. If the wind gets up, don't walk further than ten to fifteen yards from your car. Twenty yards maximum. People have been lost in white-outs. You're English and don't know these type of conditions."

'"Right. I got that." I rang off and got into my Subaru. It was a beauty of a car. It had four-wheel drive. The snow was coming down and the roads were thick with snow. The countryside was black outside. At the bottom of the hill I tried to get up the Pikey Meer twice. At the third attempt I managed.'

'What's the Pikey Meer?' asked Edward.

'It's a steep winding road which many people have crashed on or slid off,' explained Jill. 'Edward, you mustn't interrupt Mr Leasden as much as you've interrupted Dad.'

'At the top of the Pikey Meer I moved up past Gullyknowes and to a rise. I was on a small high plateau that was pitch dark. The snow was blowing across the windscreen reducing the visibility. Then I saw some small red lights in front of me. I drove up to them. It was the back of Mr Black's Land Rover. He jumped out and came to me. He was smiling all over, and didn't seem to mind a young Englishman appearing. I asked him if the road up to the farm was worse than the Pikey Meer. He said about the same. So I said I would follow him in. The Subaru would follow his tracks in the snow. He said, "Please yersel'."'

'I don't see what this has to do with Dad going out with Mum,' Edward said, yawning.

'Shut up, Ed,' said Rachel.

'Our cars drove slowly up what was now amounting to a blizzard. We had to race up the final brae to stop ourselves sliding back. Then we turned into the Followsters Farm close. Mum's dad directed me to the building.'

'Ah – Mr Black is Granda!' said Edward.

'Oh, dumbo, this is a romance! Who do you think was looking after Mum?' said Rachel.

'I went past two sliding doors which were making an awful clanking in the wind. Once inside it was quiet and warm. No wind and no snow. Tied up in the byre was a very large Charolais cow with two big feet sticking out of her end. I felt inside her and started to put ropes on the calf. Mr Black asked if we'd need help. I looked behind me. There were only two women hiding in the shadows. I said that help would be a good idea.'

'Cheek!' said Jill.

'Anyway, one of the women went for help. Mr Black and I started getting the calving ropes and the machine ready. Within a few minutes at least four large, well-muscled men had appeared. They all spoke broad Doric. I hardly understood a single word.'

'You see, Rach, me dad's a guff,' commented Edward.

'Shush, you two!' said Jill. 'A *guff* is a foreigner,' she whispered to Leasden.

'Well, we started cranking and we had a very stiff pull. If it hadn't been for those four big men the calf would never have got out.'

'I mind it was enormous,' said Jill.

'Who's interrupting now?' demanded Edward.

'Well, after it came out safely I turned round to see if anyone could help me clean my PD gown. And do you know what? Out of the dark this beautiful girl appeared.'

'Mum.'

'As a teenager.'

'I was about to go to uni.'

'Quiet in the stalls! As I say, this beautiful young girl appeared. I wondered if a beautiful girl appeared with every successful calving in Banffshire. Then they invited me in for tea. It was very pleasant. And I got a good look at the girl.'

'Did you like him, Mum?'

'Well, he was so thin! It's just like Mary said. If you take off all Dads' thick clothes there's just a scrawny chicken underneath. Your dad was very pealy-wally then. He's put on a bit of beef since. Attracted to him? Well, no. Remember he had this posh English accent and so on.'

'Anyway, my story moves on a month or so, children,' I hammered on. 'Miss Black is sitting at home with her valentine's cards. She has purchased a discount lot from the newsagents. Half a dozen at cut price. She has sent five to the real men in her life and she's stuck with the sixth valentine card. What to do with it? Throw it in the bin? She asks her mum what an earth to do with it. Is there anyone else she can send the last one too, even as a joke? Her mam say, "Why not send it to that English vet? He's probably lonely." Miss Black swithers and then decides. Why not? Game for a laugh. It will at least brighten up his day.'

'Goodness, Mam, you weren't serious!' Edward suddenly realised his genesis has relied on a massive coincidence.

'She doesn't know the young vet's first name or address. So she sends it to Mr Jones c/o of the Vets. Inside she writes, *Valentine. Remember January the fourth.* The unfortunate Mr Jones is forced to open this heavily perfumed card in the presence of the secretaries. They see the writing and the date. They rush off to the day book and identify Followsters Farm. Is there a girl there? they ask themselves. "Oh yes, there's this young quiney Black. Isn't she about to go to Aberdeen Uni?" Mr Jones is briefed by them as to who she is. So he sends a reply valentine.'

'And you would never guess what he sent me!' said Jill.

'Ah, a normal large card?' suggested Edward.

'No, this is Dad,' said Rachel suspiciously. 'Something weird, no doubt.'

'Close, Rachel,' agreed Jill.

'Mr Jones purchased a large photograph of the complete Crown Princes of Europe present at the funeral of Queen Victoria.'

'A picture of all those Princes lined up as a group!' said Edward in disbelief.

'Inside the card Mr Jones writes, "Snap valentine. I am the Prince in the back row, third from the left." Then he posts the card and soon he starts to court Miss Black. The romance begins to blossom.'

'Mum, weren't you worried that Dad was a little weird?' asked Rachel.

'Yes, I suppose so,' said Jill. 'But then I'd never met any English public school boys before, so I was expecting something peculiar.'

'Gee, I'm amazed you ever got married!' said Edward.

'Yes, I agree with you, Edward,' Leasden put in. 'It is odd. How an earth does an English/Welsh young vet educated at Cambridge go up so far north? Then how on earth does he end up marrying a farmer's daughter? Do you come from a large family?' he asked Jill.

'Well, the minister at our marriage did say he thought my family was a bit like the Mafia all over the countryside. He kept on finding my relatives in unexpected places,' explained Jill. 'I was the first in our family to get a degree at university and I'm certainly the first lawyer.'

'Amazing, isn't it?' said Leasden. 'Your parents meeting relied a lot on chance. Think, they met over the backside of a Charolais cow!'

'I'm stunned,' said Edward. 'Still, what have you got for us, Mr Leasden? Nothing so yucky and romantic, I hope.'

'Before you start, Mr Leasden,' Jill broke in. 'I think I'll lay down some ground rules. You two are not to interrupt. If you want to ask anything, make a note: there's pencil and paper handy in that box. I'm sure Mr Leasden will satisfy your curiosity later. If he needs to give you any hints before he starts, I am sure he will... Mr Leasden.'

'Thank you. This is a fable called St Brock's and the bedders. St Brock's is a college much like your school, but for older people. It is one of many that make up the University. Bedders are people who come in every day and make your bed for you. So there's no need for any student to make his bed.' Leasden thus primed Rachel and Edward.

'Now, that's what I call civilisation, Mum,' observed Edward. 'Never having to make your bed for months. This must be some sophisticated university.'

'I think it explains a lot about Dad,' interjected Rachel. 'And I think Mum would agree.' Leasden took a deep breath and began:

'In the third millennium at the old and famous University of Camford, a scandal erupted. The University comprises twenty-six colleges, full of beautiful spires and towers, with a delightful river flowing through it. In one of the colleges a bedder had been found having intimate relations with a male undergraduate student. The college was St Brock's.

'On the face of it, the fact that one undergraduate youth had gone a step too far with a college servant might have been of no consequence. Unfortunately, the media latched hold of the story and an investigative reporter, posing as an undergraduate, had been in St Brock's for a day or two. His article appeared in *The Sunday Times* and this was the first the Dean of St Brock's knew of it.

'The Dean wiped away the milk, which he had spluttered over the front page, to reveal the black print underneath: "Always on heat, the St Brock's bedders" ran the headline – this sentence purported to be a quote from one of the undergraduates.

'The next day, the tabloids joined in. An historical first was made on page three of the *Daily Magnet*. No member of the general public had ever seen the breasts of a St Brock's bedder until that day. For a fee, Samantha, the youngest college bedder, revealed all.

'She admitted that she found the undergraduates attractive, but she was going steady with her boyfriend, Sean. "Brains and balls don't always go together," she was quoted as saying. "Besides," she continued, "most bedders are older than me and able to teach the students a trick or two."

'We've had all the sex now, Mr Leasden,' remarked Edward. 'Is there any violence?'

'Shhh!' commanded Jill. 'Please go on, this is fascinating,' she said diplomatically.

'On the third day questions were asked in Parliament at Prime Minister's Question Time. MPs wanted to know, "Why is taxpayers' money being used to subsidise what amounts to private orgies?"

'One MP indicated that a constituent had written with evidence to show that in the college Corpus Albus et Niger, a college next to St Brock's, a bedder had borne a student a baby. The PM admitted that he was bewildered and had therefore called in the Chancellor and Masters of the University to see him at Number Ten that afternoon. "Obviously accidents can and do happen, but this appears to be more serious," he sagely observed; and promised to keep the House informed.

'That afternoon the Chancellor and Masters briefed the PM. Of the twenty-six colleges which made up the University, the problem was only found to be significant in four colleges: St Brock's, Corpus Albus et Niger, St Quadruped and St Meles. They promised to solve the problem as quickly as possible.'

Edward and Rachel were now scribbling furiously.

'The next day, those four colleges gave all their bedders the sack. They said the bedders would all be well compensated; but the only practical solution was to separate bedders and students. Besides, it was time the younger generation learned to make a bed as well as use it. They fully expected bedders to be allowed back in a year or two, once the problem had blown over.

'Within twenty-four hours the situation had got out of hand. The local papers had run stories indicating that many bedders were the sole breadwinners of single-parent families. Both ITV and the BBC carried the predictable news stories. There were television pictures of bedders demonstrating outside the main gates of rainswept colleges contrasted with clips of professors punting down the beautiful river on bright summer days.

'Channel Four started a series examining in detail the relevant reproductive organ parts of bedders and students. This series was designed to increase the public's general knowledge, but most people found it merely pornographic. BBC2 followed the lives of three average law-abiding bedders. This highlighted what a much maligned selection of society they were.

'"He would, wouldn't he?" said a young bedder on Radio 4. She had been told that the Masters of Meles denied spending a night in her set of flats.

'The *Daily Torygraph* had run a story indicating that ten per cent of all Camford's English undergraduates had encouraged bedders to teach them the ancient art of bundling – mentioned in Pepys's diaries.

'Furious at being so outmanoeuvred, the PM promised MPs that he would set up a high-level investigation. In the interests of common sense and objectivity, he'd have to call in a completely independent and different profession to assist.

'The next day he announced that the National Farmer's Union had agreed to supply five experienced farmers of long standing. These men not only had experience of observing *liaisons dangereuses* in the field but many had their own bed and breakfast industry experience to draw on.

'Within twenty hours the farmers' committee reported back to the PM. They reminded him of the following facts. In developed countries there was a global oversupply of graduates. While the quality could not always be guaranteed, he could always obtain more graduates at reduced cost from overseas. We lived in a global village, and research could be performed in any location from the Shetlands to London and abroad.

'Furthermore, the Internet had reduced the value of factual information; the main commodity created, stored and disseminated in Camford University. The huge subsidies paid to the University by the UGC should be reviewed. Perhaps the money could be spent in ensuring the long-term supply of food to the country. This would mean setting up an agricultural system that was free of subsidy, European involvement, completely weatherproof, less dependent on oil, ecologically balanced and s on and so forth...

'In the meantime, because of the confusion over the present problem, they had set up a five-year research programme. It would report back after the general election. Therefore, no drastic action could be taken against any one of the parties involved in the scandal. But at least the government could then be fully apprised of the facts and act objectively.

'In one single-sexed male college, all bedders would be removed for five years. Any student found having intimate relations with anyone during this period would be sacked, and the University would have to repay to him his full fees. In another mixed college, the same rules would apply.

'In the third college, all students would be double tagged and the bedders would be tagged. An automatic radar system would detect if a bedder and student were in the same room. (Unfortunately, owing to problems with the tags they were changed approximately every year.)

'Two other colleges which had never had bedders before would be forced to employ them for five years at their own expense.

'A small army of retired policemen would regularly check all the movement records of all the university students. Fines for misdemeanours would be raised against the University. The University would have to fund thee regulatory officers.

'The scandal ground on. It surfaced every time the media found little other news. Not a single news despatch mentioned any of the large pieces of quality research performed by the University. The rare research paper with dubious results always seemed to hit the headlines.

'The Prime Minister moaned to his wife that he wished people would cease badgering and pestering him on the same old story. She sympathised but did caution him not to utter those two verbs in the same breath, since it could lose him some votes. "Perceptions are so relevant nowadays," she said.

'Within two years the experiments were failing. There had been too much illicit activity. St Brock's, ahead of all other colleges, was near bankruptcy. The government decided on the advice of the farmers to cut its losses and all UGC grants were stopped. The money saved was given to universities in Wales,

Scotland, and Northern Ireland. These universities were now to perform relevant research.

'Camford University soon went bust. A hotel chain bought the buildings and made the university into a vast holiday complex, full of theme parks. The river running through the University became the prime watersport location of the UK. St Brock's was used as a training ground for bedders.

'Once qualified they worked in their own time throughout the complex. Bedders were now paid a full working wage and enjoyed a high status previously unknown.

'And the farmers? Well, that's how you know this is a fable. We all know British farmers were extinguished by academic rectitude and regulatory zeal before the year 2001.'

'That is a political story,' commented Edward, 'but still quite interesting. Can I ask you some questions, Mr Leasden?'

I got up to go and find some port, brandy or something similar.

'Were those Latin names something to do with a badger … ?'

'Are students really so sex-mad, Mr Leasden? I mean, will I be like that … ?'

I heard the questions as I left the room.

Leasden was fielding them all adroitly. It took me a while to find the necessary bottles.

When I came back there was silence. I raised my eyebrows.

'They are two very different stories,' Rachel stood up with a small piece of paper in her hand. She was acting as judge. 'The question is: "Is truth stranger than fiction?" What do you think, Ed?'

'Difficult, Rach,' Edward mused, picking at his pencil. The adults were for once silent. 'The fable was both interesting and boring. The TV and politicians are all the same all the time. So it was quite easy for Mr Leasden to make it up. But Mum and Dad – I don't see how you can make that up.'

'So?' Rachel solicited a reply.

'Well, their story is almost gross,' Edward seemed perturbed. 'I mean, I certainly wouldn't tell it to any of my friends. But Mum and Dad getting together – that's very strange, whatever way you look at it.'

'I agree,' Rachel said abruptly. 'So, Mr Leasden, you're right, you're always right. I like your story, but our judgement is that truth is stranger than fiction. Also, and I hope you'll excuse me saying this, it is often more interesting.'

Jill was shining with pride at the diplomacy of her daughter. I had to admit that she was not usually so polished in her phrases.

'Thank you, Rachel, for your kind words.' Leasden bowed his head a bit.

'She means St Brocks gets ten out of ten for effort,' Edward said, trying to be kind. Fortunately Leasden ignored any possible interpretation of sarcasm.

'Thank you both,' he said. 'I think your father has brought me some adult refreshment.'

As if on cue, Rachel and Edward left.

'They're a clever pair,' said Leasden. 'You'll need to watch them, but they could go far.'

'Thank you,' beamed Jill. 'Would you like some brandy? I think you deserve it.'

'Yes, why not.' And so the evening carried on in a relaxed fashion. Soon it was well past eleven and Leasden made his goodbyes and left.

'I like him,' commented Jill. 'I told you when I heard about him that I thought he was a real man. You know, one of those ancient chivalrous types, and yet not a fuddy-duddy.'

'Perhaps,' I said dryly.

'You're jealous!' she expostulated. 'I can see it.'

'That is a no-win position for you to take,' I countered, 'and you know it.'

'Deny it, then!' she demanded.

'I deny it,' I said. 'I am a vet, he is a teacher. I do; he tells how to do. I rest my case.'

'I'm not sure I believe you.' She examined my face and then looked away. 'Still, let's be like Pepys. A man your teacher mentioned.'

'Ugh?' I was lost.

'"And so to bed…" Bundling, anyone?'

I followed her up.

Chapter Fourteen

Naturam expelles furca, tamen usque recurret – If you drive nature out with a pitchfork, she will soon find a way back.

Horace, 65–8 BC

It was the beginning of the day. I opened the door for Leasden and he went in. He didn't move far inside but set his stocky body to one side, looking at a man who was pushing his head through the reception window.

'There is no need to stamp these bills with "Overdue" in red,' we heard coming out from the office over squat swarthy shoulders clothed in rough old tweed. 'You'll get your monies. That I promise you. It's even written in my will: "Settle the vet's account before the funeral director's account." Trust me, I've been with you many years. Too many, perhaps.'

'Oh, I am sure that's not true,' June smiled and handed him his cheque to sign. She had worked with the building societies for years before coming to us, and so was almost immune to pleadings about money. She once confided one of her greatest thrills was to become calmer and calmer while someone lost their rag more and more. 'It's all in the building society's training manual,' she had told me.

'Well, whatever,' he queried. 'I hope not to see you for a while. The feeling is perhaps mutual?'

'Oh, not at all,' said June, smooth and calm as a cool drink. 'We're always happy to see you.' By now the pungent odour of a pig farm had hit me. Even Leasden was sniffing, moving his grey head around in an attempt to find an air space which was breathable. That last sentence from June was to my mind a lie. (I later accused her of this false statement. 'Not if he has money,' she had said triumphantly.)

'Well, good day, madam.'

'*Miss*.'

'Pardon, miss.'

He turned around to face the door and we caught sight of his countenance in full: a tweed pork-pie hat with a bit of dust and chaff in it; a round face with sideburns which unmistakeably gave the impression of the cheeks of a boar; large bristling eyebrows and slightly red face with steel-grey eyes completed the face. A solid sixty-year-old man, possibly an ex-scrum half.

'Gooday, vit'n'ry,' he said to me, and touched his hat and exited.

A mud imprint of a piece of the tread of his shoe was left on the doormat. June rushed out of the office spraying air-freshener into the waiting room. Leasden raised his eyebrows; he often seemed surprised at the company I kept.

'Well, that was Mr McCann. He has a croft and a pig farm – as you no doubt guessed,' I informed Leasden. I thought no more of it and we commenced a typical day's work.

That evening I was on duty. About ten p.m. the phone rang. Jill answered it and looked very nonplussed. She covered the headset.

'I'm not sure who it is. It makes no sense, but it's not English.' In her mind a significant percentage of my fellow countrymen from south of the border had mental deficiencies. 'Actually I think he's drunk. You had better see if you can get some sense from him. Keeps on going on about why he never pays his bill.' I took the phone.

'Is that you, vit'n'ry?' I heard a slightly slurred voice about to commence a diatribe and no doubt checking it had a target in its sights. I had a fair idea what was coming.

'Yes, it's me – Richard; we met this morning, briefly,' I said. It sounded like Mr McCann. 'Mr McCann, isn't it?'

'Yes, thank you, sir. And that is my point: why I do not pay my bill.'

'Oh?' I said, nonplussed.

'As soon as I pay my bill and we are all square then you buggers want to come and drink from my cup again. Always wanting to drink from my fountain!' McCann slurred a little. I thought I could just detect the muffled sounds of a pub behind him. I let him carry on. 'Now, less than twenty-four hours later I need you to come out to see my sow. She stuck in pig – farrowing, I mean. Just my damned bad luck. More bills. You'll come now, please.'

'Oh, so you have a sow stuck farrowing and you need a hand?' I attempted to confirm some reality.

'Yes, that is correct, you have it in one,' said the voice at the other end.

'Where are you, Mr McCann? If I go now, will you be at the farm?' The sounds of the pub concerned me.

'Never you mind where I am!' I heard sniggers in the distance. 'You or a colleague leave now, and I'll meet you at the farm. Millfield – you know it?' he shouted at me.

'Yes, that's no problem. One of us will be there soon. Bye.' I put the phone down. Jill looked concerned. It had not been a normal conversation.

'Oh, it's just an old boy. A little upset about needing us again so soon. Plus a little drink, I think. His family will be there. Mrs McCann is fine.'

'Well, you just be careful what you say,' Jill also thought most Englishmen like me too bumptious and useless with country manners in delicate situations.

'I will, I will.' I knew what she was getting at.

I drove off into the dark. The wind was gusting and the car wobbled occasionally. Now and then a little rain came down as well. It was pitch black. I arrived at the farm and stopped well short of the farmhouse, which stood in front of me. It was a solid old-style building. It had a slightly bent roof with a few slates loose. A single phone line ran away from it. The wire was gyrating in the wind. It was highlighted by one single light set on a pole above one of the low buildings on my left. The pole was shifting, causing the shadows to be constantly on the move. The wind grabbed my car door as I opened it and a great gust of cold air rushed inside it as the internal light came on. I got out and faced the low building, on my right. It joined up with all the other buildings all the way to the house. The top of a half-heck door was open and I could see inside a naked light bulb illuminating a series of farrowing pens. I turned briefly to look at the rest of the close. No sign of human activity, just dark puddles reflecting the intermittent light. It was hard to hear anything above the constant gusts and the creaks of the ancient farm buildings.

'Mr McCann!' I shouted. 'Mrs McCann!' No answer. Inside the farrowing area there were sows looking fairly contented. One, lying down, had a little clear discharge from her rear. 'Well, that's the patient,' I said out loud, if only to encourage myself. I poked my head over the half-heck door and looked at the house. There was no sign of life, though with a closer look I could see a flickering light produced no doubt by a coal fire. 'Oh,' I said to myself. 'Oh dear.'

Then I heard the sound of human speech. A kind of mumbling noise coupled with the sound of uncoordinated feet going through the puddles. Weaving his way into the court from the direction of the track came Mr McCann.

'That you, vit'n'ry? My, you are fast! These modern cars, no doubt.' He came toward me, swaying.

'Is this the one?' I asked.

'Aye, aye,' he replied.

I grabbed some kit from the car, put on a long green PD gown and bent down behind the sow. She was nestled in her farrowing crate. All the time McCann had been following me with his eyes fixed on my face.

'Can we close the top of the door and put that light on, please?' I said.

'Sure.' He quickly turned round and looked at me close. I could hear that he was speaking to me in as sure an English accent as he could manage, with few hints of Doric.

'I don't recognise you. You look very young.' He said this as if accusing me of being on the run.

'I just don't wear my glasses at night. I am long-sighted and see better at night without them. We met this morning.'

'I doubt it.' Now I caught a terrific blast of alcohol from his breath.

'You very young. Perhaps this is virgin territory for you.'

I looked at the rounded pale buttocks of the sow and the pink vulva and grimaced.

'Not virgin territory for her,' he carried on. 'Of course, she has pigs. How long were you at university?' I was just beginning to insert my hand inside the sow. I stopped and considered. Better tell the truth.

'Eight years.'

'Eight years! My God! You must be lacking in brains. My goodness, and they sent you here to me tonight!'

'No. You see I was at Cambridge. We do two degrees there. That takes six years, and then I studied tropical vet at Edinburgh for two years. So eight years.'

'So you're like a pop group – three degrees!' he laughed at his own joke. Then looked seriously at me. 'Why such a long time studying for tropical medicine? It's a long way from this farm in Inverden in Scotland to Africa. Only if you travel at speed of light able to do a farm visit. Speed of sound is too slow. You made a mistake there.'

I couldn't fault his physics, but needed to get on with the sow. He saw my look. I put my hand in and felt all to be normal. A piglet was just there waiting to pop out.

'Have you let her have any oxytocin?' I queried, with my head now quite close to the floor.

'Ox toes, oxtail?' he said, looking at me. He appeared bemused, leaning on the top rails at the farrowing crate, contemplating my prone position. 'No, I have never given any of my sows ox; not natural at all.'

'No,' I remembered Jill's plea and took a deep breath. 'Oxytocin – it's drug … it helps them push.'

'That may be what you call it,' he said, 'but I think at other universities they call it pituitrin.'

'Yes, yes that's it,' I said.

'No.' Pause. 'I ran out.'

'Okay, it doesn't matter. I'll give her one shot now.'

I turned round. My gown covered me like a large curtain. I found some oxytocin and injected her. Then I put my hand in and extricated one piglet. It was alive and well. I put it up towards the sow's nipples. She grunted in quiet acknowledgement.

'It will go well?' he asked.

'I think so.'

'Good.' He straightened himself up and put his hand into the deep left pocket of his long overcoat. A small miniature of whisky emerged. He unscrewed the cap and was about to drink and then saw me. He raised his eyebrows and proffered it.

'No thank you… driving, Thanks for the offer.'

'It's nothing. I feel sorry for you driving. Perhaps next time get a driver.'

I pulled another two piglets out as he shoved his hand deep into his right pocket. A bottle of strong stout came out.

'Chaser!' he said. And he knocked the lid off against one of the horizontal farrowing crate bars. He lifted the bottle up and emptied it in one. Then he turned to me and belched a slow, quiet, satisfying belch. I could see him trying to focus in my direction. My hand was deep inside the sow, my chin against her rear. But he wasn't looking at me.

'My, my!' he said beaming. 'Six piglets already! You may be young but you're a damned good vet. So fast!'

I paused and wondered whether to tell him the truth: there were as yet only three. Then I remembered Jill's request. There was no point being a clever clogs now.

'It's good,' I said, my voice absolutely neutral. Three more quickly came out and made their way to the side of the sow. They were amazingly quick at finding a teat. Two rows of six teats lined up on the sow.

'Och, that is brilliant! Twelve living, and they look so lively! Twelve is a reasonable litter.'

I continued on, and quite quickly had another six out. My tray of equipment was to my side and I searched around for a syringe and some antibiotic to give the sow. This would lessen the risk of a womb infection. I was just sinking the needle into her when I heard him say, 'Twenty-four! Well, that is excellent. I've had that number once before, of course. But never so lively and large.'

Sitting back on my haunches I saw twelve very healthy-looking piglets all well attached to the teats. It was a pleasure just to sit and watch them all happy in the glow of a lamp, sucking away like crazy. I collected my thoughts, took a breath and said, 'I'll just check her one more time.' As far as I could feel, and the womb of a pig is very long, there were no more piglets. 'I think that's it.'

'Of course it is, of course it is,' said McCann. A huge drunken smile settled on his face.

With my kit in my hand I stood up, and turned round. McCann went ahead of me to the door. As he went over the doorstep he swayed and almost fell over. Quickly I put my kit down and went to him.

'Vit'n'ry, help. I'm weak on my legs. Could you please help me into the house. I am sorry … You gather I phoned you from the pub. Drown my sorrows. Only joke – I have no big sorrows!' He was looking very unsteady.

'That's no problem,' I said, and with the left shoulder of my PD gown (which was clean) I supported him. He immediately transferred a lot of his weight to me, almost clinging to me. We moved forward slowly. 'The family are not here?'

'No, no, they all went to a film, full of blood, violence and murder. I said I wasn't going to no such thing. Enough in the real world, why do I need more? I was in Korea: hell of a time. Film called *Road to Purgatory*. Well, well, I'm on the stairway to heaven. A little drink, a little help from my vit'n'ry friend, and oh my! A lot of piglets healthy.' He stood up straight with effort and looked at me. 'You understand real life?'

'Yes,' I said, determined to avoid a philosophical discussion at all costs.

'Good, good. Real life is full of jokes and sadness. For instance,' and here he leaned on me with some weight, 'someone could think that you and I are two homosexuals much in love. Here we are hugging each other.' He sniggered

'That has an element of humour,' I said cautiously.

'Don't you worry. I am straight, vit'n'ry. Four children straight, one each year, then stop. My tackle is fine: it goes straight when I see attractive woman, not man. I prefer women to men. No, I rephrase that: I only prefer women.' We lurched forward again.

'Oh, don't worry,' I said seeing as he was in confiding mood, 'I've been in an English public school. Done that bit; got the medal.'

'Quite, quite,' he said, as if he completely understood. 'It is a teenage thing. Not for now, no, no, not now.'

He belched a halitotic and alcoholic vapour at me. I smiled diplomatically and looked around at the dilapidated farmyard. The wind rushed around my ankles, a little chaff blew in my face, water from the roofs occasionally came down and caught me on the face... It was cold and drear. He was right, I mused. Even if I was a rampant homosexual, the time, the place and the person were all wrong for a quick act of sodomy.

'Almost there,' he said, as we waddled the last few yards to the house. We stood at the door. The wind appeared to freshen as we got there. McCann pushed his hand down at the handle. The door opened a couple of inches and he inserted his hand to find the light switch. With his bottle he pushed the door wide open and almost fell down inside. In doing so he pulled me in quickly after him. With my spare hand I closed the door. The room was very cosy and warm in a sort of tweedy, old-style way. The coal fire on the left was still alight and beside it was obviously his chair – a large chair with its cover darned and repaired many times. No doubt it had a solid frame. Some pillows and a blanket were in it.

'Help me to the chair, please.'

I guided him over. He reeled around, facing me, fell back and collapsed into it.

'Are you okay?' I said. He looked not too bad. My long PD gown was casting shadows all over the room.

'Vit'n'ry, you look like some caped crusader. Course I'm fine. I want you to do three things for me.'

'Yes?'

'First, do not tell the family where I been tonight.'

'Fine, no problem.'

'Second and third: put some more coal on the fire and remove my shoes. I have bad arthritis and it's very hard for me to do that.'

'Sure.' I pulled of his boots and laid them in a place on the edge of the hearth. Then I took away the fireguard and built up the fire. Once the fire was set I looked up. McCann was completely out. I stood up and fished in my trousers. There was a roll of peppermints in my pocket. I placed it in his lap. One brief look and all appeared safe. I hurried out, slammed the door and checked it was secure. He wasn't going to wake for a while. Then I walked purposefully across to the farrowing house. Inside I retrieved my kit and examined the sow. All appeared fine. I cleaned my boots by the tap, The wind raised my PD gown up so I took it off and got back in the car. It was time to head for home. What a man, I thought.

It was quiet and all the lights were out when I got back.

'Richard, is that you?' A voice came down from the floor above.

'Aye, yes. I'll be coming to bed soon.'

'What happened?'

'Oh, I'm not sure you'd believe me if I told you.'

'You never tell me anything.'

'That's not quite true. Anyway, I often think you would find it all boring or a fiction. Then you might think I was carrying on with someone else.'

'You are ridiculous!'

'Besides, it was a little unreal.'

'So you say.' I climbed up to the voice upstairs.

The next morning I was in the office when the phone rang.

'Mr McCann for you, Richard. He said, "Please whisper."'

I frowned and took the phone.

'Yes?' I said

'Ah, vit'n'ry,' I could hear McCann speaking quietly. 'Can you help me? My wife and I cannot understand something. My wife cannot understand how I told her that there were twenty-four piglets when this morning we find only twelve. It's very strange.' I heard a click and guessed that Mrs McCann had joined the conversation by an extension.

'Well, Mr and Mrs McCann,' I said, trying to give the old boy a hint, 'it does sound strange, but cannibalism is not unheard of. She may have eaten them. Usually they go on till there are none left, but as an adult she may have stopped, particularly if she is happy with her normal food this morning.' I was beginning to put in a little veterinary fiction.

'Yes, she is eating well this morning ...' broke in Mrs McCann.

'Is that you, Mother?' said Mr McCann in surprise.

'Well, hopefully that'll be the end of it. As long as the food's okay she'll be fine,' I went on.

'Oh good, good! Vit'n'ry, you are clever. By the way, thank you for the mints: my wife says for the first time she can smell the difference between my head and my tail.' He laughed

'Robert Dominic Thaddaeus McCann, how dare you be so coarse! What an embarrassment – and to a professional man.'

'But it was you who said it, Mother!' I heard him plead.

'Yes, but not for all to know... Really, what you get up to when we go to the cinema, I don't know.'

'I can assure you, Mrs McCann, that both your husband and I were responsible and did the best possible for your sow,' I butted in.

'I'm sure you're right – and I am glad you came, Mr Jones. Yes, of course I am that. The farm after all is the most important thing,' she said, mollified.

'Well, vit'n'ry,' interpolated McCann, 'thank you! You are a wise man for such a young head. Goodbye.' And the phone went dead.

'What on earth was that all about?' demanded Neil.

'Oh, if you have a spare ten minutes I'll tell you. But don't worry, it's all in hand and as far as I see under control,' I replied.

'McCann?' queried Neil.

'Yes, but I think it's okay,' I said. Then I completely forgot about it until about five days later when Leasden and I were returning from a call.

'Base to Vet Three, over,' went the radio. I turned down the Wagner we had agreed to listen to.

'Yes, what is it?'

'Can you go to McCann, Millfield? He has a sow that he's unhappy about. Mrs McCann phoned.'

'Okay, we'll go there now,' I replied and turned up the Wagner again.

'Isn't that the farmer last week who wasn't too keen on paying bills?'

Leasden doesn't miss much, I thought.

'Yes, it is the very one. He's a funny old boy. But don't worry; Mrs McCann is there. She brings reason to the situation. She is a good old soul.'

At this stage I didn't want to fill Leasden with all the whys and wherefores.

We arrived in the close. There were two young teenagers loading a wheelbarrow when we arrived. At the same time, Mrs McCann, grey-haired with a simple headscarf, duffel coat, skirt and wellies, came out.

'They look young children,' said Leasden.

'They'll be the grandchildren. Two of their sons work on the rigs, another is a bobby in Liverpool and the daughter is married to a local bank manager. With their dad on the rigs they quite like to spend time on the farm; it's a good education.' I thought I'd get this dig in. So many children nowadays had so little sense. One reason seemed to be their lack of first-hand knowledge of nature or farming.

'Quite, quite,' said Leasden. It was water off a duck's back to him.

We got out of the car. The close looked a little brighter today, though the mud was still jet black and damp. Mrs McCann came toward us, a smile in her face.

'I am glad you've come, Father is worried about one of his sows. Just farrowed … Now she's not eating at all and I am sure she has a fever.' She held her hands together.

'Not the one I farrowed?' I asked with some concern.

'No, no, she is doing fine. Mind you, one of her piglets was crushed but the other eleven are doing fine.' She smiled a weak smile. Then McCann pushed his head out of the half-heck door. He rotated his head one way and then the other and settled his gaze on me.

'Vit'n'ry! Come in here, and bring your father too.' I was about to explain that Leasden was not my father and then shrugged and followed him into the farrowing house.

'There she is. See – very sad, the little piglets looking for milk. I doubt she has any.'

We congregated around the farrowing crate. The sow was lying flat out and breathing a little heavily. She grunted a little and looked back at us out of the corner of one eye. Her food trough in front of her was full and obviously untouched. The piglets were running up and down her teats, trying them. McCann was right; there probably was no milk. The pigs were still fat and had clearly been getting some nourishment until quite recently, so I reckoned we might be in with a chance. I bent down to take her temperature.

'It's a good thing you called me so quick. These piglets have not been starved too long; if I can get an antibiotic that can work, we may save the litter yet,' I informed him. The fear is always that you can save the sow but she stops producing milk for so many hours that the piglets die of starvation. Cross-fostering was risky; you needed a suitable sow in milk, and feeding them by hand was a high-risk strategy. There was a discharge coming from her. She had a temperature and the mammary glands were firm. The little milk I could find appeared normal.

'She most likely has this condition MMA – mastitis metritis agalactia. I'll give her an injection, and you can follow it up with some jabs in the next few days.'

McCann looked stunned at my pronouncement. He turned to Leasden. 'Are you also a man of learning?' he asked.

'Oh, yes, and I am not his father. *Agalactia* comes from Greek. Something I know well. Possibly better than Mr Jones.'

Amazed, I wondered where this conversation was going to go. Then I relaxed. If the conversational equivalent of Ulysses and King Kong were going to meet, then fate had dictated it so.

'Oh, so you taught Mr Brown! He told me he took eight years to qualify. Was he lacking?' McCann let it hang there.

'In some areas of course. I doubt without a dictionary he could have explained what *mastitis*, *metritis* and *agalactia* come from—'

'Ah, there you all are. What have you done?' Mrs McCann, having disappeared temporarily, had come back to restore sanity to the situation.

'Vit'n'ry's about to treat sow,' said Mr McCann, realising he had strayed from the job in hand.

'Ah yes, Mrs McCann, since she has farrowed so recently I think it worth a try to flush out the womb. Can you help me? I need to fill a calf stomach tube bag with an antibiotic solution.'

She and I could handle the practicalities with speed. We went to the farmhouse after I had grabbed a calf feeder from my car. Leasden and McCann were left in conversation with one job to do – inject the sow. I had given them a loaded syringe. Mrs McCann and I mixed the antibiotic powder in some water in a clean bucket. The calf feeder consisted of a long, blunt-ended tube about two or more feet long. It was fed fluid by a plastic bag, which one held up vertically by the top of the bag. At the bottom of the bag the tube joined it. There was a snib on the tube for blocking off the fluid until the tube was in the correct place. When we had it ready we returned to the farrowing house.

'I never knew how important Latin and Greek was to medicine,' said a beaming Mr McCann. They were obviously getting on like a house on fire.

'Did you inject her?' demanded Mrs McCann.

'Oh yes. Professor Leasden did it, just like that. With force! No messing about.'

I looked at Leasden suspiciously; he shrugged his shoulders.

'Definitely in the beast?' I asked.

'*Oh yes,*' they chorused.

'Good,' said Mrs McCann. 'Now, Father, you come here and help. Mr Brown is going to insert the tube inside her. I'll open the snib and you hold the bag.' She held up the now taut and full wide tube-shaped bag while I bent down behind the sow and gently inserted the tube up the womb. It went in very neatly.

'Here, Father,' said Mrs McCann. Without looking she passed the bag to Mr McCann beside her. Mr McCann grabbed the bag by the base and not the top. The column of fluid in the bag, now having no support from the top, collapsed over on one side and emptied its three pints over my bent head and shoulders.

'Oh, Father! What have you done?' was all I could hear as I lay transfixed under the deluge.

When I got up I saw Leasden turning away, his whole body quaking with laughter.

'Quite!' I stood up, water pouring from me. As a southerner I was determined to retain my sangfroid. The top half of my body, including my inner vest, was soaked.

'Ah'm sorry. Such a mistake,' remarked Mr McCann, looking genuinely surprised.

'Oh, these things happen, even with the best intentions,' said Leasden, trying to make Mr McCann feel better about his blunder.

My jaw dropped. He had never been so conciliatory to me in the classroom. This behaviour amounted to hypocrisy.

'Still, we must give this treatment. Let us try again.'

I turned to Mrs McCann. Together we walked out of the building. We were back in a few minutes. This time we succeeded.

'You must get home right away,' encouraged Mrs McCann. 'Change yourself quick and out on some dry clothes. I could give you some of Father's but I think they are not suitable for a gentleman like you.'

'Yes, I think we had better go.' Leasden and I hurried to the car. 'Give me a phone to tell me how she and the piglets are doing, won't you?'

'Of course, of course,' she said hastily. 'Now, you get along there now.'

We drove off. Leasden was silent and I was beginning to feel chilled. He was obviously holding himself in since there was the suggestion of a grin at the corners of his mouth.

'If you don't mind, I will drop you off here at the practice,' I murmured. 'You can tell them what occurred.'

'Righto.' Leasden rolled his stocky frame out of the car seat and moved to the office.

I turned the car round and headed for home. Fortunately there was some hot water left. The best solution in these circumstances was a hot bath. It was a joy. After only two minutes in it the phone rang. Still in the bath, I managed to answer it.

'You okay?' It was Neil.

'You heard?'

'Yes, your friend told me.' He laughed a little. 'But I was still a little concerned. Sometimes these things are worse than they seem.'

'Thanks, Neil. Yes, I'm fine. I'll be round in a minute or two.'

'No, that isn't why I phoned. There's nothing new here for you. We'll see you when we see you.'

Neil knew that when something odd happens it is often better to let your colleague gather his thoughts and come back to the fray on his own terms. It is, after all, what I would do to him.

Half an hour later I was back and we started another round of calls.

The pattern of rural life is such that disasters or significant events often occur in threes. So it was no surprise to me to be phoned around seven thirty one morning by Neil.

'If it rains it pours,' he said. I was up and half dressed. No doubt Neil sounded upset. Perhaps he wasn't going to get his swimming.

'I've just had McCann on the phone. Evidently one of his sows has just torn herself at the end of farrowing. Probably some piglet's sharp teeth when it came out. It sounds like she may have also ripped herself on the rear of the farrowing crate. That's his fault for not maintaining it and taking the sharp edges away.' I wondered why I was getting this blow-by-blow account. 'Anyway, he demanded that you and "the professor" come out now. He was panicking, saying there's fair amount of blood. I told him I would come out as I am on duty. He didn't like that. It told him we couldn't stand and argue on the phone while the pig was bleeding. He said he had seen blood come faster. "Send the professor who speaks Greek." I shouted at him he needed a surgeon, not a Classicist. Jesus! That was a mistake, shouting, I admit. He just started ranting and raving. Mrs McCann must have been outside. Anyway, he said he'd let me come, but would only pay if you did it. And then he rang off.'

'Okay, okay,' I said. 'But we'd better not make a habit of this.'

'Well, if it makes you feel any better, the phone rang immediately after. Someone desperate to get through after McCann's blathering. It was McCutcheon – he has a heifer with a five-day dead calf inside her, he thinks.'

'Oh, fair dos, Neil. I'll take McCann.'

'I thought you would,' said Neil

'I can go myself, can't I?' I said.

'What? Oh ya, sure. Leave Leasden. Keep it simple. Just go and stitch the sow up. Must go. Cheers.'

'Cheers.'

I reversed my car out of the yard and almost ran someone down. It was Leasden.

'I thought you'd be asleep!' Leasden stated, standing stock-still while I unwound my window to check he was in one piece.

'The impression is mutual.' It was not my intention to give way to his domineering probing.

'Anything interesting?' he queried. I paused. To tell the truth or no? Better just bite the bullet.

'Yes, get in. Your fan, Mr McCann, was hoping you would accompany me to a bleeding sow. Unless you have any massive objections, you'd better fulfil his wishes. Besides, with you present we stand a better chance of getting money from the old sod – for some bizarre reason which I cannot fathom.'

'Fine by me,' said Leasden. And off we went.

On arrival at the farm the usual suspects were there.

'Nice to see you, both of you,' said Mr McCann. 'I'm afraid we have no light in the farrowing house. It'll take me some time to fix it. In the meantime my grandson will hold one torch and, Professor, can you please hold another? Mother will stand outside and pray. Only a joke, Mother! Have you got all your stuff?'

'Yes, thanks. Lead on, please.'

We all bent our heads down and trooped in through the half-heck door to the farrowing pens. The scene was cinemaesque, with the torches only illuminating along their narrow beams of light. Little light reflected off the walls. The pigs were like huge pale ghosts. There was a dripping noise and the sound of our feet in small puddles. For a pig house it was all eerily quiet.

'One of the puddles is of blood,' advised MrMcCann. 'I think it's the next sow up.'

Our group of huddled bodies shuffled slowly on. Sure enough we had found the sow. She had ripped her swollen vulva on the sharp back of the crate and at the same time Neil's guess had been correct – the piglet's teeth had probably torn the last third of the vagina. There was a fair amount of blood lying in a small pool. On closer inspection there was one arteriole spurting. That single vessel was probably the cause of nearly all the blood. It might even stop itself, given time. But now I was here it would be better to tie it off and stitch her up. I opened the back of the crate and once again found myself behind a sow. Leasden put my tray of instruments and medicines beside me. I gave the sow a sedative to take the edge of her, put in some local and placed a single clamp on the bleeding vessel. Then I began to prepare the operating site.

'If you stand to my left,' I said to Leasden, 'and your grandson, Mr McCann, stands on my right and shine your torches down in the area, I will have enough light to work in. You must sort out the sharp bits on the rear of this crate as soon as you can get some light, Mr McCann.'

'Sure, sure, the grandchildren and I will do that,' said McCann.

I began to clean and disinfect the rear of the sow and prepare my instruments, suture thread and swabs. Soon all was ready: a clean operating site; all surgical equipment to hand; and a stationary animal.

'Is everything okay?' shouted Mrs McCann from far away at the door.

'Perfect!' I shouted back. 'We're just about to start.' I picked up my forceps and suture needle with a needle holder and was just leaning forward when something whistled past the front of my nose. A partial eclipse had occurred. Only Leasden's light shone. The reason why became obvious in the reduced light of one torch. The grandson had fainted and buried his mouth and nose in my clean operating site. All I could see was the back of his head, flanked by the two buttocks of the sow.

'Bugger!' I said.

'At least that,' said Mr McCann. He stood stock-still.

'What's happening?' shouted Mrs McCann in the distance. She could detect something untoward, even from far away.

'Don't move, Leasden – keep the light there,' I said. I knew he'd be tempted to move the narrow beam of his torch and so leave us in darkness. I needn't have worried too much. Mr McCann bent down and with the typical latent strength of a farmer effortlessly lifted his grandson up. He turned him round and put him down against the wall.

'Stupid boy! He never has breakfast, not even a piece and tea. Then of course he keeps on fainting when there's something like this.' McCann turned round to face us. We looked at him. He looked back at us.

'Shouldn't you check him?' asked Leasden.

'No, no, no he's done this many times. But to please you, shine a light on him.'

Leasden did. The boy was propped against the wall and breathing regularly. His hair was tousled, his face was covered in blood and the tip of his tongue could just be seen. In the uncertain light the innocent grandson's relaxed face gave an appearance consistent with a young cannibal sleeping off his first orgy.

'He's fine,' said Leasden. No doubt he had had many faint in his classrooms before. In his case it would have been induced by sheer terror.

We returned to the job in hand. Mr McCann held the other torch and the sow let me complete the job.

'My, my, quite neat,' observed Mr McCann. 'Do I have to take the stitches out? Any other treatment?'

'You can take them out in about fourteen days if you want; but they will dissolve themselves in about four weeks. I'll leave you some injections for the next few days or so,' I replied.

The grandson started moving and blinked. He looked very sheepish. He knew exactly what had happened.

'Now look here, Robert,' explained McCann. 'You're very lucky you fell on something soft. One day you could hit your head and damage what's inside. What is inside is precious, probably better than what is inside my head. Ask the professor here!' He indicated Leasden.

'Yes, it's precious stuff,' agreed Leasden. We stood in a semicircle round the young man.

'Now, you promise me this, Robert. From now on you will always have breakfast or at least two slices of toast and some tea before you come out on the farm with me. Got that? If you agree – and I have two witnesses here – then I won't tell your grandmother.'

As if on cue, a voice outside shouted, 'Father, what are you up to?'

'It's all right, Mother. We come out now and then I'll fix the electrics. Robert, promise me?'

'Yes, Granda, I promise I will.'

'Fine, fine.' McCann tousled his grandson's head. 'Come, let's go, these are busy men. They have work to do.'

We all emerged into the sunlight and blinked. Leasden and I tidied ourselves up by a tap.

'Cheerio, Mr McCann. I think that's your three. Won't be seeing you for a while now,' I volunteered.

'Yes, I hope you're right. That is three quite enough for now.' He smiled, certain in his own mind that his luck would change.

'What was that all about?' asked Leasden as we drove away.

'Oh, it's one of the patterns of life... rather like the Gulf Stream, or high tides with the new moon. For a farmer, bad things – which include calling the vet out – always occur in threes. He's had his three, so that is it.'

'You don't believe that, surely?' He eyed me with suspicion.

'In fact it's a really good rule of thumb,' I replied blithely. 'I didn't credit it much when I first came. But now I've been here a few years I find it's a bit like the seasons: part of the pattern of rural life. Sure, you get unseasonable weather now and then – two disasters – but normally it goes in threes.'

There, I thought, I've silenced him. And I had.

Chapter Fifteen

Aequam memento rebus in arduis servare mentem – Remember when life's path is steep to keep your mind even.

Horace, 65–8 BC

'Who's on duty tonight?' asked June.

'I think Richard has that pleasure,' Anne answered.

'Aye, aye,' I said. We were all in the office at the end of the day.

'Right, I'll switch these phones through,' said June. She dialled the ★ button followed by 21★ and then my house number followed by #. Putting the receiver down, she took a few paces to her left and picked up the handset of the fax machine. June dialled the practice number.

'Is that you, Jill?' she checked. 'You've got the phones. Richard's coming down now.'

A couple of minutes later I had arrived home. My feet made a scrunching noise as I headed for the garden gate. Once along the path, my gait was silent. As I passed the bow window I glanced in briefly, expecting to see the usual moonlike shapes of teenage faces gazing at the TV. Instead I saw them reading. I paused for a second and noted that their heads were bent down, each concentrating on a paperback. I sniffed in disbelief and went into the kitchen.

'Busy day,' I said.

'Well, so was mine,' came the retort. 'Supper is almost ready. I'm going to call the children.'

'Yes, what are they up to?' I asked.

'Reading – hadn't you noticed?' Jill told me.

'Okay, but what are they finding so gripping?' I followed on. 'Did you ask?'

'I didn't want to disturb them,' said Jill. She paused and then a typically feminine explanation came. 'But then I did ask.'

'And?'

'Oh, they both said "one of the classics". So I left it at that,' she explained. 'I reckon your Classics master has set them onto the classics. Great, isn't it? My pun isn't bad either. But then you wouldn't want to acknowledge that.'

'Are they my books?' I asked.

'Oh yes, they said they had worked through your books and the ones Grandpa passed on to you,' she explained.

'Oh well, miracles never cease,' I said. 'At least I hope that is the case.' To my mind something didn't quite fit.

The phone rang.

'Inverden Vet Centre?' answered Jill. Frowns had crossed both our faces. The tension had increased a little. Someone was giving Jill a long explanation. She listened, cocking her head waiting for a break in the monologue.

'Thank you, I think I had better hand you over to the vet.' She passed the phone to me, whispering, 'She says it's urgent,' and then raised her eyebrows.

'Hello. I am the vet,' I stated. 'How can I help?'

'I am sorry to bother you,' commenced the explanation. 'I'm Mrs Fiddes of Theak Avenue. My Rory is awfa sick. He's weak and wobbly in his legs and I think he needs a vet soon.'

'What is his main sign? His weakness?' I asked.

'Na, it's diarrhoea with blood in it. I think that's what's making him weak. Though it might be his heart. He's only about six year auld.'

'How long has he had the diarrhoea for?'

'He's had it for at least four days, and I was hoping and hoping it would clear up. But now there is blood in it I'm feart I could lose him. My sister checked him today during morning and the afternoon and said he was in some pain. So as soon as I came back from work I phoned you for help. Rory is straining a lot too.'

'Well, it may be his straining for four days which has caused the blood. Perhaps he should have seen a vet earlier,' I gently chided her.

'Well, can you come round right now?' she asked.

'In fact it would be better if you came round to my surgery now,' I countered, not wanting to be wandering round a housing estate where all the numbers were jumbled up. 'Can you manage right now?'

'Ooh, now is it that urgent?' A note of surprise came into her voice. I took a deep silent breath. 'I mean I'd have to get my neighbour to drive me. My man isn't back yet.'

'Well, I'm free now,' I explained. 'I might get called out at any minute to a calving or something similar as an emergency. Can you get your neighbour to bring you round?'

'Okay, I am sure I can, vet,' she agreed. 'I'll see you in five minutes, right.'

'Right, look forward to seeing you,' I said and put the phone down.

'She's an awful blather, that lady,' commented Jill. 'She gave me a great scree about Rory and his motions and how weak and tottery he was getting.'

'Aye, aye. Supper will have to be on hold for me.' I put my head round the door. 'Rachel, Edward – supper.' They trooped in.

'We'll eat now,' Jill told them. 'Dad is off to see a dog.'

'Bad luck, Pops,' Rachel was sympathetic. 'What's worst with it?'

'Four day-old diarrhoea with blood coming out now. Gotta go.'

'Rachel, did you have to ask? How can I eat now?' an irate Edward ranted at his sister. I left.

The surgery was in darkness as I turned in and drove round the back to park my car. I walked round to the front. The pale white lights from the street reflected off the puddles in the old car park tarmac. Two locks had to be released before I could get in. Then I switched on more lights, and looked for a white lab coat and the correct record card from the files. I heard a scuffling noise outside. It was peculiar how at out of hours visits owners made this distinctive scuffling noise in the surgery porch. One day, I thought, I will analyse it. During normal working hours they just walk in bold as brass. Out of hours and the characteristic scuffling noise is to be heard. I cut to the chase and opened the door.

'Come in.' I stepped aside. 'Come in, come in, please.'

In came Rory, a Jack Russell terrier. He was prancing on his own tip-toes. His little tail was wagging in a fast but different rhythm to his tongue, which was popping in and out of his mouth. He was a picture of bright, alert interest.

'My, my, the fresh air has done him so much good,' chirruped Mrs Fiddes, a stout smiling lady. 'It's almost as though we don't need the vet now after all.'

I gave a weak smile and showed her the door to the consulting room.

She gloried on. 'I hope I haven't ruined your tea. I just missed your closing at six I see, by the notice at the door.'

'No,' I said calmly. 'I'm usually able to pick up food somewhere along the line – learnt that in the cadets.'

'Good, good. Mind you, it's so hard to get anyone these days; fortnight to see a doctor, you know. You vets are so easy and helpful.'

I looked at her and wondered how many of her ilk had quite thoughtlessly ruined the marriages, family lives and driven to drink or suicide the veterinary surgeons of this country. For a second I paused and took full stock of this smiling being standing in front of me with a prancing terrier beside her. And at that moment I realised that she and her fellow selfish creatures were either unaware of the mayhem they caused or were in complete denial.

'Well, I'd better check him over,' I said brightly. I was damned if I was going to give her the slightest satisfaction or hint of the discomfort she produced. She whipped Rory onto the table. He froze. I came close to him and saw the corner of his mouth tremble and his gaze fix dead ahead. I had seen that look in Jack Russells many times. Before we went any further I realised we had to clear something up.

'Does Rory bite?' I asked. 'Has he ever bitten anyone before?'

'Rory? Rory has never bitten anyone, Mr Jones!' She stroked him. 'No, never, ever.'

'Oh, that's fine,' I said, and approached him with confidence. As my hand came close to his body the little flicker in the corner of his mouth changed to a full growl and he whipped his head round and snapped at me. Years of practice and the early time of the evening meant that my hand retracted away in the nick of time. All one could hear was the clop of his jaws meeting.

'I thought you said Rory had never bitten anyone?' I asked, a little perturbed.

'Yes, that is correct,' she smiled. 'The darling has tried many times but he's never actually bitten anyone – at least, not hard. Most vets tie his nose but I thought you might be special. So I let you carry on.'

'Well, I am an ordinary mortal,' I let on, deadpan, 'so Rory is to be tied up.'

This I did. Mrs Fiddes winced and tut-tutted. 'Don't worry, Mrs Fiddes, I won't hurt him,' I said. 'All I have to do is my normal checks.'

A few minutes later I had checked there was little wrong. I gave him an injection of vitamins, some medicines to bring back normal gut function, and then I untied him.

'Thank you, Mr Jones,' she said.

We moved to the office. I informed her how much the consultation would be.

'Oh, I'm not sure I have enough,' she told me. 'Can I pay tomorrow?'

'Sure,' I said. 'I'll just make a note in the book.' Just then a head came round the door.

'Hey, Nancy,' uttered the head, 'give me your bag – I need to get some fags, and Willie is needing some books from the lottery!'

Mrs Fiddes did me the grace of blushing a fraction.

'Off you go!' She gave away the bag. Her words came out with surprising harshness; then, as she turned to me, they regained a more syrupy flavour. 'Come on, Rory, say bye-bye to that nice young vet, Mr Jones.' They sailed out into the dark. Slowly I exhaled. The temptation to take up smoking is never so real, I thought. Thank goodness that little terrier had not made a mess of my hand. There are some people who think their pet 'having a go' at the vet is a bit of fun.

'Let's go back to the pleasant world,' I said aloud. I phoned Jill. 'Anything doing?'

'No, can I put on your tea?' Jill asked.

'Good idea,' I said. Soon I was back home.

'I'm sorry but it's only spaghetti Bolognese,' Jill said. 'I was too tired to do more, and it's been reheated in the microwave.'

'It's fine,' I told her. Edward entered.

'All okay with the dog?' he asked.

'Yes, but I'm not sure you want the details,' I said. 'Might unsettle you.'

'No, it's okay, on you go.' He sat down at the table clutching his paperback.

'How's the reading going?' Jill was in her usual inquisitive mode.

'Fine, Mum,' he replied. 'Sometime I could give you a taste of it.'

'Why not now?' she carried on. Rachel had entered.

'Don't think it's appropriate,' Edward murmured. 'Rachel would agree, not when Dad is eating. We both found the same book. One is dad's copy, the other Grandpa's.'

'Edward's right,' said Rachel. 'Laters.'

'If it's one of those classics,' Jill pressed, 'then Dad won't mind, I am sure of that. They are, after all, his books.'

Edward looked at Rachel and said, 'Very well, Mum. You asked for it.' Jill turned to the washing in the sink while Edward cleared his throat.

'... And at the window out she put her hole,
And Absalon, so fortune framed the farce,
Put up his mouth and kissed her naked arse
Most savorously before he knew this.
And back he started. Something was amiss;
He knew quite well a woman has no beard.
Yet something rough and hairy had appeared.'[2]

I put down my fork.

'What the f—ck is that?' said Jill, turning round, her face incandescent.

'Jill,' I said. 'Language!'

'Language, language, you – you Richard!' She was nearly shouting. 'Did you hear what our son just read? That was excrement!'

'It *is* a classic, Mum,' interjected Rachel. 'I can vouch for that. Edward and I found them after Mr Leasden came.'

---

[2] Chaucer, *The Canterbury Tales*, translated by Neville Coghill, Penguin Classics, 1957 reprint, EV Rieu series editor

'Listen, there's more,' continued Edward. 'I think it rhymes if you listen carefully.' Unperturbed, he went on.

'Now Nicholas had risen for a piss,
And thought he could improve upon the jape
And make him kiss his arse ere he escape,
And opened the window with a jerk,
Stuck out his arse, a handsome piece of work,
Buttocks and all, as far as to the haunch.
Said Absalon, all set to make a launch,
"Speak, pretty bird, I know not where thou art!"
This Nicholas at once let fly a fart
As loud as if it were a thunderclap.
He was near blinded by the blast, poor chap,
But his hot iron was ready; with a thump
He smote him in the middle of the rump.'

'Richard, is this your Mr Leasden's doing?' Jill demanded.

'No, I think you don't get it,' I countered, 'do you? It may be your fault.'

'My fault?' She was surprised and stood up straight. 'Look at Rachel – she's glued to it. What have you got, Rachel?'

'Mine rhymes too,' Rachel said. And acting all innocence, she launched into it.

'Alan rose up; and towards the wench he crept.
The wench lay flat upon her back and slept,
And ere she saw him, he had drawn so nigh
It was too late for her to give a cry,
And in a word, they very soon got on.
Now Alan, play! For I will speak of John.
John waited for a while, then gave a leap
And thrust himself upon this worthy wife.
It was the merriest fit in all her life
For John went deep and thrust away like mad
It was a jolly life for either lad…'

'Dear,' I said, trying to break it gently. 'It is not Burns. This is Chaucer. It is a little your fault.'

'My fault!' She was shocked. 'How come?'

'Do you not remember going on about the classics when Leasden was here? Don't you remember you mentioned Chaucer?

Leasden rather abruptly said, "No – go for Solzhenitsyn." Well, the children smelt a rat and made a beeline for Chaucer.'

'Yes, Mum,' said Rachel. 'Thanks for your suggestion … catch a load of this!' She intoned:

"'Well, then, reach down your hand along my back,"
The sick man said, "and if you grope behind,
Beneath my buttocks you are sure to find
Something I've hidden there for secrecy."
"Ah," thought the friar, "that's the thing for me!"
And down he launched his hand and searched the cleft
In hope of finding what he had been left.
When the sick man could feel him here and there
Groping about his fundament with care,
Into the Friar's hand he blew a fart.
There never was a farm-horse drawing cart
That farted with more prodigious sound.'

'Sorry dearest,' I said. 'They win. Still, it's possibly better than a PlayStation 2 manual.'

'I can give you my manual to read, Mum,' said Edward, 'if you want something clean to read.'

I frowned at Edward and nodded him to leave the room.

When they had gone Jill sighed.

'I don't know how to educate them,' she said. 'You try and try, and still it's like hitting your head against a brick wall.'

'Don't worry,' I said. 'We've probably got the basics right. They do speak to us. They even try to read some of our books.'

'Oh yes – the filthy ones,' she said. 'Mind you, I did some Chaucer at school. I don't remember it being as crude as that, thrusting and so on.'

'Well it shows they're better investigators than we were,' I said. 'Don't worry, they will be fine. The language is in fact quite good. Or let us put it this way; there are some good turns of expression. Come on, love, let us have a cup of tea and rest the brain watching TV.'

The rest of the evening Jill and I lounged on the sofa idly watching the screen. The inevitable phone call seemed to have disappeared into thin air. I was in that pleasant frame of mind where the brain is hardly engaged and doesn't care. Odd snatches of poetry came to me. Jill was leaning against me and I knew I would soon be dozing. The *Song of Songs* rose to my mind: 'Blow on my garden that its fragrance may spread abroad... Eat, O friends and drink, drink your fill, O lovers...'

The phone went. For a flicker of a second a set of emotions welled up. Jill passed me the phone.

'Hallo, Richard? It's Duncan here. Sorry to disturb you so late.' I could hear Duncan's distinct timbre.

'That's okay, Duncan. Problems?' I asked.

'Afraid so. I have a heifer stuck at the calving. Could you come?' He knew I would, but still he had the grace to request me.

'Aye, aye, sure,' I said. I knew he wouldn't phone unless he had just cause. 'I'll just get myself ready and be up as soon as I can.'

'Fine, thanks.' The phone went dead.

The emotions returned. How unfair this was, everyone else was having a good time. What other folk at no notice had to go out solo to solve a problem in such an exposed manner? As a matter of discipline, I rejected these thoughts and quickly turned my mind to steel. The modern jargon would have miscalled this 'positive thinking': I found that too unrealistic. This was my job, and that was the glory and the shame of it.

'I've got to go,' I said to Jill. 'Come to think of it, I'll make it easier for me and take some company. I'll give Leasden a buzz; he said he wanted to see some of the emergency work. Now is his chance.'

Jill gathered a blanket to her to compensate for the sudden loss of warmth. 'You will do no such thing. He's retired, Richard, show some sense.'

'He's pretty fit,' I retorted. 'I think he is up to it. It was his idea.'

'But up Duncan's hill? I heard that call. Leasden may well have friends or relatives back at Norbury. You're not to damage him,' she urged me.

'He has relatives ... as for friends, well, I don't know,' I sniffed. Jill was anxious for some reason. I couldn't fathom it out. 'Look, honestly I'm sure he'll be fine. No problem.'

'Well, you be careful with him,' she said firmly. 'Bring him back in one piece.'

'I understand that it is the beast I am off to save,' was my double entendre parting shot. I phoned from the kitchen to avoid more uxorial ire. Leasden sounded interested, even excited.

'He's keen to go,' I shouted to the sitting room.

At the square I picked him up. He was properly clothed for bad weather and rain. Jill needn't have worried, I reflected.

The farm was miles away high in the hills. We drove in silence.

We entered the square of the next village. All the street lights were on. In the middle of the square stood the statue of a soldier guarding the names of the fallen of two world wars. That was the only human shape we could see. At that point I turned off the main road, drove away out of the lights of the village and up into the hills. Leasden did not know, but on either side of us stood great hills. Soon we were level with some of them and the lights of the village which we had passed could be seen down behind us.

At the farm I parked my car by the farm buildings and we got out. I noticed opposite me, on the other side of the small road, a field gate uncharacteristically open; it was as though it was beckoning me. I stepped back to the building, peeked in and saw no one. On turning round I saw two dark silhouettes walking towards us. The farm lights behind them hid their faces.

'Oh, hello, Duncan Andrew,' I said, recognising their outlines. 'I've got Mr Leasden to give us a hand if necessary. Is she in here?'

'No, no, she's up on the hill.' Duncan pointed upwards into the pitch black where I knew the hill to be. The open field gate now beckoned me like the opening to some vast chasm.

'Oh, we just go in there and up the hill to her!' I tried to be light-hearted.

'Yes – we tied her to a digger and tried to calve her with the machine. But she went down and it became surprisingly stiff. So I thought I'd get you.' Duncan was matter-of-fact. At least he hadn't irritated me by using that awful phrase – 'So I thought I'd get the expert'.

I paused. Leasden looked at me. I needed some honest replies.

'Truthfully, Duncan, is it possibly a Caesar?' We were all experienced and I didn't want any dodging the issue.

'Likely,' he said. Our eyes met.

'Right, okay fine,' I said affirmatively. 'We need at least two buckets of clean water and some torches. This is a challenge. Can I get my car up there?'

'Oh yes,' Duncan replied. 'I think you can. Neil drove his car in that field. You just go along the bottom of the field and then up.'

I wondered if Duncan knew that last week Neil's car had at long last been traded in for the miraculous sum of £1000. It had not been worth a tenth of that.

'Right, I'll give it a try,' I said. 'She's that end of the field halfway up, isn't she?' I pointed into the void on my left. Duncan nodded and returned to the house for the water.

It was around the time that Elgin, not eighty miles away, had been comprehensively flooded not once but twice. The field was very wet, and the car pitched and yawed as we progressed across the grass. Out of the corner of my eye I saw Leasden's head go down almost to his knees and then curve back to the headrest.

'I'm not sure Renault designed this car for this,' he commented.

'I agree,' I said, 'but it's a good car all the same. The wheels are wide and give some grip. Tell you what, I'll try to cut across to the heifer.' I began to point the nose of the car up the hill. The nose wobbled back and forth, sweeping the field with the beams of the car. Suddenly the wheels gripped. The car spun round as I wrestled the steering wheel. We saw the nose veer round, point straight up the hill and then curve back all the way round past the lights of the faraway village onward down to the farm lights and finally to the bottom of the field. Leasden saw an angled vista of the Highlands at night quickly sweep before him. I braked.

'Perhaps we'd better follow them,' I said. I could see the lights of Duncan's four-wheel drive bumping along below me. We slid down to their level and found a reasonable track.

'Cognescenti of the hill,' murmured Leasden as we saw them suddenly turn right and head directly up the hill along a firm path. Soon we could make out the lights of the digger flickering out into the night.

Right enough, the heifer was down and pressing. In fact she was making a good effort of it. The headlights of Duncan's car illuminated her. She was a few yards down the slope from the digger, and attached to it by a halter.

I got out and felt inside her. Although she had managed to push the forefeet well up and had the head well into the pelvis it felt tight. The calf's nose was sticking out a fraction from the vulva. Laterally where the calf's elbows were, there was very little room. On the ventral floor of the pelvis there was no room to speak of. It was likely that if we did pull it out the forces used would crush the chest. The calf was still alive.

'You gave it a pull?' I double-checked with Duncan.

'Yes, but it got very, very stiff.'

That all tied up with the elbows of the calf and the narrow hips of the heifer. Although the pull had potentially endangered the calf's life, the calf stood a better chance if we Caesared the heifer now.

'Okay – it's a Caesar,' I said. 'We will have to make the best of it out here. Hardly ideal conditions.'

'Oh, I don't know,' chipped in Andrew. 'It is dry now. There's been no here rain for few hours. Best do it before the next shower.'

'Aye,' added Duncan. 'It's not too bad.' I could sense they were joshing me.

'You mean we are lucky on this hill not to be working in blind drift with the threat of a touch of hail,' I laughed.

'That's about it,' said Duncan.

'Can you hold her, Duncan, while I put the sedative and womb relaxant into the vein at the neck?' I asked him. I moved forward with a head torch on. Just as Duncan approached her she got up. He quickly took the halter and brought it tighter to the digger.

'Let her lean back, Duncan,' I said. 'Often when they try to reverse it highlights the jugular well. As long as she doesn't come forward suddenly I'll be okay.' I bent down in front and slightly to one side of the heifer. I found the jugular and injected the drugs. 'Okay, let's slacken the halter a little,' I instructed. Then I returned to the car and began to prepare my two trays of kit. Leasden held the torch. I got in the car and turned it a little to put more light on the heifer. Duncan did the same with his four-wheel drive. The heifer went down. She had gone down on her left side, so we rolled her over to lie on her right side. Duncan and Andrew tied her feet up and pulled them to the digger at the front and my car at the rear. Leasden and I placed the trays behind us and began to prepare the heifer. We injected her with local anaesthetic and then cleaned her side. A drape was placed on her. Andrew and Duncan stood the other side of the heifer from me.

'Tell you what, Leasden,' I said, 'could you sit on the heifer's neck to keep her down? Just sit on the topside so as not to obstruct the windpipe. You'll get a good view from there; if you're bored you can look at the all the lights of the different towns below. Andrew, you come round and give me hand. Just wash your hands in this bucket here and I'll then put some alcohol on them.' They all changed places.

The operation went on as normal. The air was fresh and dry. Soon we had the calf out. Andrew and I rushed to the digger and hung it there for a while. It began to breathe.

'Looks good,' I said. 'Andrew, keep it there for a minute more then put it down somewhere safe and we'll get on.'

I went back to a bucket, cleaned my hands and started to remove as much placenta as possible from the womb. Andrew rejoined me and held the womb while I sewed it up. A torch went out and Duncan replaced it. Soon it was all done. I completed my checks.

'Are you okay, Leasden?' I asked.

'Couldn't be better,' he commented. 'That was fascinating.'

'Well, you can get off her neck now,' I said. 'She'll get up sometime soon.' Leasden started to help me pack up. We tried to walk in the beams of the car lights. The wind started to get up and it became a little chilly. The calf had moved itself under the digger and was shivering.

'Are you going to take the calf in tonight?' I asked Duncan.

'No, I don't want to,' replied Duncan. 'I'll give it colostrum now. Don't worry.'

'Well, you know your beasts,' I said.

'It's shivering, which means it's keeping itself warm,' explained Duncan. 'Besides, taking into the buildings risks it getting an infection. It might start scouring or get navel ill.'

I couldn't argue with that. I only hoped Duncan knew about his beasts. 'We will be on our way, if that's okay by you,' I said.

'Sure, but you're welcome to come in for some tea and to clean-up,' said Duncan.

I swithered. Better get home and tidied up there.

'Thanks – better dash. It's getting cold. Cheers. Keep in touch.'

'Cheers… thanks, see you.'

Off we went. The field was ever bumpy as we lurched into the road. Its smoothness caused us both to relax. We headed back to Inverden.

'What's that?' asked Leasden.

'What?' I slowed down.

'Wait, it has gone.' Leasden appeared bemused. 'No, there it is again in the sky.' I peered and saw a glimmer I recognised.

'I think it's the Northern Lights.' I was uncertain. 'It is usually very cold when they are out. Mind you, the temperature has been going down and it's still clear. Oh yes, I have just seen a big display. That's it.'

'*Aurora borealis*?' said Leasden.

'Yes, have you never seen it before?' I asked.

'Never, no, never. It's amazing, almost supernatural.'

'In that case you had better get a good look at them,' I said, and stopped the car in the middle of the road. I switched off the headlights and left the sidelights on. 'It's okay. You can do anything in a road in the country provided the others can clearly see you from a great distance. This is the middle of a long straight. Go on and have a look.' Small flashes of light moved across the sky.

Our eyes accustomed to the darkness above the dimmed lights of the car dashboard. We could discern more stars every minute. The sky was not after all pitch black but had a blue tinge to it. Suddenly, flashing curtains of light lit up most of the northern horizon. This curtain began waving and bending as though ruffled by some breeze. A second or two later it shot over our heads and disappeared. It was quickly followed by another curtain of light. Although each had a common shade of green and moved to a similar rhythm, their size and shape differed. Some occupied the whole sky, while others took up fractions of the horizon.

'We can't see it clearly like this,' I said. 'Better get out.' We both moved out of the warm cosy cockpit of the car and stood in the road leaning on our opened doors.

'Incredible!' said Leasden. I looked at him over the top of the car.

'Oh, do you believe in God?' I asked without thinking. I almost bit my tongue off at my indiscretion.

'Oh, yes,' he replied. Then I remembered I'd spotted him outside the church when Aunt Sarah and I had left. 'With good reason,' he added. 'And you?'

'Yes.' I reminded myself that there always had to be reasons with him. 'And your reasons?'

'They boil down to about three,' he said, his head cocked up high at the sky. 'You see, I am a Classicist. I have read copies of nearly all those old manuscripts in their original languages. The manuscripts of the New Testament are very well authenticated, at least compared to any other old manuscripts by, say, Josephus or Julius Caesar. More importantly the style of these gospel writers has a ring of truth to it. After you have travelled through Livy or Herodotus you finally come across these books and they are like a breath of fresh air. Mark has a breathless immediacy while Luke is detailed and lively. Unless you have read all these authors it is difficult to describe, but the Gospels are vibrant in comparison to many other Classic pieces. Even Plato's conversations are stilted by comparison and the Greek comedies are lively but unreal.' He paused.

'And your second reason?' I queried.

'Ah well, there seems to be good evidence for the supernatural in the Gospels. By that I mean it seems to me that the resurrection did occur as an historical fact.'

'How can you say that? Whoa!' I whispered as four sections of the sky lit up with colour.

'Well, put it this way, how could you describe this display of the Northern Lights to someone who lives in the jungle near the equator? You've been in the tropics. How would you describe this illumination above us to someone who might well disbelieve you?'

'I'd try my best to be accurate and reasonable. I would also seek to have other witnesses to back me up,' I replied.

'You will find something very similar in style in the Gospels. They know they are describing something or someone supernatural. They do just what you said; they emphasise accuracy, reason and corroborating witnesses.' I understood Leasden had thought this through.

I searched the sky, drinking in the beauty. It was very quiet and cold. It would be tricky to describe these Northern Lights to anyone in Africa, I had to admit that. They might well think I was mad.

'Your third reason?' I asked, looking over the top of the car to Leasden, who was still gazing up to the sky.

'Ah, the third is more to do with heart than style and reason,' he confessed. 'Perhaps you know the opening to John's Gospel: "In the beginning was the Word and the Word was with God, and the Word was God..." Now that is a magnificent opening. It is like that of a great symphony or massive drama. It suggests that the heart of God is very large and tender...'

'Leasden,' I interrupted. 'You are a romantic, really!'

'No, no, that same passage not only has those magnificent phrases but also delicate and loving ones: "There was a man sent from God his name was John." And, "He came to his own home, and his people received him not." Or even, "The light shines in the darkness, and the darkness has not overcome it."'

'And from that you deduce that God has a large heart?' I said. 'You may be correct, my favourite from John is, "There is no fear in love, But perfect love drives out fear." But I don't understand the large heart you mention.'

'Well, yes. Big-hearted in the best sense of the word, like a father,' Leasden followed on.

'Well, perhaps I can go some way along with that,' I concurred. 'But what about suffering?'

'The Son of God who loved me and gave himself for me,' explained Leasden. 'You can look at all the massacres and pogroms of the world described in history books and yet you see he came down from his position of power and pogromed himself, for our sake.'

'You mean he met it head-on?'

'Yes, and he didn't have to. Why didn't he leave our galaxy to rot? It is rotten anyway.' Just then some tremendous flashes of the lights blotted out the stars.

'Aye, you have a point,' I said. 'Still, I reckon to have been fortunate; nothing so bad as that has happened to me… probably the same for you.'

'Yes, no seismic disasters – one bitter event, that is all,' he said ruefully.

'Oh?'

'My wife died in childbirth with our first child,' he said plainly. 'It was hard to take at the time.' I wondered if that had made him so severe. As if divining my thoughts he went on, 'You may find it hard to believe, but that softened me somewhat. I became less severe, took a more long-term and relaxed view after that.' Embarrassed, I decided to change the subject.

'My, it is cold. That's the problem with these Northern Lights – it's always so cold.'

'Which is why you never saw them in the jungle – or perhaps my physics is astray.' He seemed relaxed again.

We got back into the car. I dropped Leasden at his hotel and thanked him for his company.

'He is back safe and sound,' I said to Jill as I went up to the bedroom.

'*He*, I hope, being Leasden?' she asked.

'Of course,' I said.

Chapter Sixteen
At the cutting edge

Leasden, Emma, and I were sitting in reception, each in a different corner, facing in and chatting. There was little happening. The phone had gone quiet. Neil was out testing a herd and Anne was next door sorting out some small animal drug orders.

A woman appeared opposite the sliding glass window of the office and stood facing us. Being the nearest, I rose up and moved the window across.

'Are you a mixed practice?' she enquired.

'Yes. We do all species that are presented to us. How can I help?'

'Well, do you do anything?' she asked. At this point I examined her closely. Her hair was perfect, not a single fibre out of place. She was about late thirties, dressed in dull rural clothes which were spotless. There was no clue in her appearance as to her background.

'That is an odd question. But yes, we do anything provided it is a veterinary matter, not illegal, and you are satisfied with our work for you. What had you in mind? Mrs er...?' I fished for her name.

'Mrs Semple. You won't think I am mad, will you?' she smiled. By now I knew this conversation was well inside the boundary limits of uniqueness.

'Excuse me saying so, but you don't look mad. So why not tell us what you had in mind?' Leasden and Emma were listening in attentively. 'Is it a job for a vet?'

'Oh, yes! Definitely. In fact, according to the scientists only a vet can do it. So if I want this done I have to find a willing vet.'

'It is?' I asked

'Well, I hardly dare to mention it. In fact my husband thinks I

253

am a little touched. But I used to live out in Medley Croft. We left it two years ago and now live in the States. We still own the croft but are about to sell it. So that's why I want to act now.'

'Fine,' I said, completely lost.

'We had two dogs when we lived in the croft. They were great friends but when they were put down because of illness we had them buried in the garden at the croft,' she explained.

'Go on,' I said. By now I had gripped the low desk in front of me and was pinching it hard.

'Now, I am in contact with an American firm. They say if I can obtain a piece of the dog's tissue they will preserve the DNA. When the technology comes along they will be able to clone the DNA and reproduce our two dogs. It sounds weird, but I really would like to try,' she continued breathlessly. 'I work, so my husband said I can spend some of my money on this if I really want. He said he would help only because he cares for me. He thinks we should leave them alone.' I had some sympathy with the husband but also knew people could become closely attached to their pets.

'I don't see where a vet comes into this?' I said in genuine bewilderment. She frowned, so on a more positive note I continued, 'However, what I can say is that I hope you've thought through the implications. I'm not offering you counselling, but you have to realise that even if this did work out, the dog you then would have, while genetically identical would not be your original dog. That is why twins are genetically identical, but two different people.' I tried to check how much of a grip of reality this lady had.

'Yes, yes, I have thought all this through. I know it's a long shot, but I don't see why anyone should stop me trying,' she said.

'I agree with you completely there,' I replied. 'There's nothing unethical in what you want to do, and if it's your wish and within your power and you are not hurting anyone else – go for it.'

'Good, I am glad you said that. You have put my mind at rest. You have been very helpful.'

'Glad to be of help,' I said, and assumed that was all the help she required.

'Now, I need a vet,' she said, 'and I think you and your colleagues may be able to help me.'

'How do you mean?' I asked.

'The company in the States, Newlife Bionics, insists that the samples taken from the dogs have to be taken by a veterinary surgeon. You have not refused. So I would be grateful if you could help me. I will of course pay for your services,' she explained.

'What exactly is it that you want us to do?'

'Well, you should come to our croft on a day we agree. My husband will dig up the graves and all you have to do is open the boxes they are in and take the samples, put them in the correct containers and send them by courier with the completed documents. The company will make sure the documentation is fine for import/export. If you agree I will ask them to send the pack to your practice address.'

'I tell you what,' I said, 'could you just give me your contact telephone number? I'll speak with my partner to see if we can do this. I will phone within twenty-four hours.'

'Sure.' She frowned again and doubt crept into her voice. She wrote the details down and left.

Leasden and Emma were silent. They had seen nothing like it before. A few minutes later Neil appeared. I explained the matter as best as I could to him.

'Come down the back, Richard. We'll discuss it there.' Neil turned down to the back of the surgery. 'I don't see why she needs a vet for this,' he commented, once I had shut the door.

'Oh, it is in the what's-its-name bionics company's protocol, I gather.'

'Well, we are short of money this month. We could do with some more funds. The question is: is this a type of business we should be getting in to? It's a little too close to bodysnatching.' Neil rubbed the sole of his shoe against a step.

'It isn't at all,' I countered. 'The owner *wants* us to tamper with the body. She is the legal owner. I don't see any legal problem at all.'

'Yes, Richard, I know the croft. I even know of her. The croft is not sold yet; that I do know.' Neil had all sorts of contacts in the countryside who kept him up to date with all the local business. 'But is it ethical? When you qualified, did you think this was something you would be excelling in? What would you think of another vet who did it? Just for money. Is money everything?'

'Neil, she needs a vet to do it. We provide a service. I don't think she's asking us to do anything immoral. Granted, it was not what I thought I would be doing when I qualified. But that holds true for a lot odd things I've done since I qualified.'

Neil snorted and kicked the step. 'That's true enough. Ye Gods! The things we have had to do to in this age to earn a crust. Okay, you set it up, and take Leasden with you.'

'He said he wasn't going to come. He mumbled something about teaching a dead language and not needing or wanting to be involved in a canine necropolis,' I replied.

'He's lost me.' Neil looked bewildered. 'Well, can you manage yourself?'

'No, Neil. If this is to be done then you and I will have to do it. I couldn't ask an assistant like Anne to help.'

'So… so…' Neil stared at me. I met his gaze. We both looked deadpan. Neither blinked for a couple of seconds. Then Neil moved.

'Okay – what you are about to do, do quickly.'

'Neil, that's what Jesus said to Judas,' I chided him.

'Yes, yes, quite. I may take it back. We'll just have to do it. It is complete madness. But she will definitely get a vet to do the deed and so it might as well be us. This must not get out.' He looked up to the door to the office. 'Tell the staff: news blackout!'

'Right, I'll get going on it. If you want, I could phone the Royal College in London to double check on the ethics?' I suggested. This was an attempt to make him feel more comfortable.

'No, don't contact them. First they would not give a straight answer, second they would launch an investigation or some such rubbish. Much better they don't know. It is a long way from Inverden to London.'

'Righto, just leave it to me. Don't worry, it'll be okay; besides, there is no one else I would prefer to do this job with than you,' I said.

'Thank you for your vote of confidence! Just make sure we have time and are not hurried.'

I left Neil pacing up and down. He reminded me of someone

on the point of delivering 'To be or not to be'. Back in the office I instructed the others about the need for complete secrecy until a decent time after the event. Then I phoned Mrs Semple.

'I have spoken to my partner and we agree to do it for you,' I informed her.

'Oh good, good!' She sounded excited. 'I thought you wouldn't come back. You seemed so serious.'

'Well, it is a serious matter.' I kept my voice deadpan while I grabbed the table top to pinch it again. 'We will try to do a professional job for you.'

'Great!' she said. 'Look, I'm going to phone the company in the States now and I'll ask them to send the kit to you as soon as possible by courier. It will have all the instructions inside. You must make sure you have prepared for the specimens to be sent back within twenty-four hours of obtaining them.'

'Right, I'm sure we can manage that,' I answered. However, I didn't see the need for the urgency. Both dogs had been dead for well over two years.

The next day much to my surprise at lunchtime a small courier parcel appeared. Inside were all the instructions with all the requisite import documentation to complete. That was easy enough. Then I checked the four vials we had been given. Two for each dog. A sample of bone marrow, or skin or lymph tissue had to be placed in a tube. Neil and I discussed the matter. We thought after such a length of time that the lymph tissue would be difficult to spot. Bone marrow and skin was feasible. Leasden listened for a while about our recollections of trips to the knackery on which we based our reasoning. He blanched and left us to it.

'Well, that's the first time we have found your academic friend not up to it,' Neil remarked, noting Leasden's absence. 'He is usually able to face anything, but we have seen him off with this.' He sniggered a little.

'Yes, but we still have to face these dogs, Neil. I think we had better hide our glee until after we have done this,' I cautioned.

'Right enough,' Neil became serious again. 'Have you fixed a time?'

'Yes, this afternoon. Anne is free to cover for us if any calvings come up.'

'That's pretty fast, Richard!' Neil parried my urgency.

'It was you who told me to be quick, remember?' I said quietly.

'Oh, Yes… yes… so I did.' Neil swallowed. 'Right, this afternoon it is. We will go in my car, bring all your tricks. I'll bring the post-mortem stuff.' I turned to the phone and contacted the courier.

We needed them to come and pick up the specimens first thing the next morning.

'Where are you exactly?' the technician asked.

'Inverden in Banffshire,' I volunteered.

'Oh, I can't see that anywhere at all.'

'It's in Scotland.'

'Still can't find you on the computer's location finder.'

'Well, we are on the mainland.'

'Oh really? I can't find you anywhere. You'll have to give me your postcode.'

'BA45 7HP.'

'Oh my goodness. I have you now. My, my. You do live in an obscure part!'

'It's not that unpleasant.'

'No, of course. Silly me. Right, now I've set the computer on that location we'll be with you at nine thirty tomorrow morning. Is that okay for your requirements?'

'That is fine, thank you.'

'Everything okay?' Neil demanded.

'Yes! Extraordinary, that man. He thinks we are in an obscure part of the country. Ramsay MacDonald came from near here, and the famous author MacDonald, of CS Lewis fame, also hails from this part of Britain.'

'Some of your countrymen are so ignorant I feel embarrassed for you,' Neil kidded me. 'I wonder what primary schooling they receive.'

'You might be correct.' I decided to placate him. 'Though in my defence, some of my primary schooling took place in Malaysia. Well, I'm off for lunch. We meet at two forty-five.'

At two forty-five I settled down into Neil's car. His dog Malc was on the back seat staring at my neck. I had usurped his seat.

'I know where the croft is – just enjoy the ride,' said Neil, who seemed to be in an uncharacteristic mood of bravado. I leant back and closed my eyes. Heavy breathing started up by my right ear. Malc was letting me know I was in his place. He was a large and good-natured Labrador, so I ignored him. Sooner rather than later I heard Neil say, 'Right, here we are.'

I opened my eyes; there was little to see. A har had come in from the coast. We were in thick fog. Straining my eyes, I could make out the edge of a low bungalow about five yards away.

'Just the weather for it,' murmured Neil. We got out and walked to the house. Mr and Mrs Semple emerged out from the mist.

'You found us,' she said. 'Well done! My husband has done nearly all the digging, so just come round.'

We followed the two by the side of the house into a small garden. It was surrounded by a small conifer hedge. At the far end there was an alcove of grass. The centre of it had been dug up. Neil and I approached. We stood by the graves. A little further on were two headstones marked 'Brandy' and 'Snap'.

'Aha, a sense of humour!' stated Neil loudly. 'The names, I mean,' he added, in case there was any misunderstanding.

'Oh yes,' said Mr Semple, nonplussed. To him it was obvious this was no laughing matter.

I looked down into the grave and saw two oblong boxes about three feet down. A small brass plaque on each gave the name. Neil got down in the grave with Mr Semple who had a jemmy, screwdriver, hammer, crowbar and chisel wedged in his large fist. Together they began to open the lid of Brandy's coffin. The screwdriver did most of the work. Mrs Semple gazed on transfixed. I stood by, nursing the sample containers, labels, and plastic bags which would soon be required. The weather had now become extremely mild and dull. We had torches to hand to help us see in the gloaming. Swarms of large midges started to appear. Fortunately they were not biting midges. Attracted to heat, they not only circled around the torches but also began to gyrate towards the two men sweating away down in the grave.

Neil slowly and ceremoniously removed the lid. Mrs Semple did not move. I peered down. It was a sight new to me. The dog was in a damp mummified state. Thin yellow-grey skin was fixed taughtly over the skeletal frame. Most of the hair had gone, though a few tufts were present, reminiscent of a dog with severe mange. The eye sockets were empty. Neil's face showed no emotion. He bent down and sized up the situation.

'Right. I will crack this bone here, which is obvious and easy to get at. I'll get a sample of bone marrow from that. The skin is easy to do. Pass me those two.' He indicated a bone saw and some other bone surgery items. I passed them to him. 'Just stay there, Richard; I'll manage.'

Deftly, Neil cut into the bone. 'Now, Richard, pass me the forceps so I can get the sample and lower the sample tube down toward me.'

This I did. I held the tube close to Neil's site of operation and was just about to open the lid when we were halted by a deafening shout. I jumped and almost finished in the grave but regained my balance in the nick of time.

'Stop! Stop! Don't put an insect in with Brandy! I only want Brandy!' Mrs Semple had suddenly come alive from her transfixed state. Neil and Mr Semple hardly moved but just looked at each other. I had the distinct impression that they had met many women like Mrs Semple before.

'It's quite okay. I will be careful,' replied Neil quietly. 'There are a lot of midges around, but don't worry. Besides, Richard will check the tube.'

Down we all bent. Neil very quickly grabbed a piece of dusty bone marrow and popped it into the tube. I examined the tube with the torch. All it contained was the tissue. I smiled at Mrs Semple, and before I could do anything more Neil was at me.

'Ready, Richard.'

Quickly I bent down with the other tube. In went a sliver of moist skin. Neil had been careful to take a full thickness piece so as to obtain the germinal layer for the bionics company. By now the midges were out in force.

'I think you are right, Mrs Semple. The midges are terrible – can we sample somewhere else?' suggested Neil.

'Yes, that's a good idea. There's an old veranda in the back of the house. We could put the coffin of Snap on the coffee table.'

'Good, I think that would be wise,' said Neil.

Now, although we had all agreed the course of action, its execution left me with a sight I will never forget. Neil and Mr Semple lifted the coffin of the dog out of the grave. It was heavy and must have been designed for a dog about the same size as an Alsatian. Then in the dull light of a Scottish winter's dusk, they lugged the coffin toward the building. The mist was still swirling around. The coffin was followed by Mrs Semple holding the torches, while I came in the rear, carrying jemmy, screwdriver, hammer, crowbar, chisel and all the veterinary kit. What, I wondered, would anyone think if they ever saw this procession?

Neil and Mr Semple put the coffin down on the coffee table. The torches revealed an old sun lounge with a few soft chairs. Their covers were riddled with holes and the stuffing was beginning to appear. Cobwebs hung from the ceiling corners. Dead insects littered the floor. It was getting darker. Neil and Mr Semple attacked the lid again. It opened up to reveal an enormous dog. I saw Neil blink, step back and swallow hard. It was as though all his bravado had left him. He gave me a stunned look and said, 'Oh, I've got to do something. Richard, carry on, I'll be back sometime.'

Immediately, he disappeared. My jaw dropped. Mr and Mrs Semple's eyes followed him and then turned back to me. This had not been in my game plan. What was Neil up to? I fully expected to hear the car fire up and hear him drive away.

'Well?' she said softly.

'Ah, yes, well,' I reiterated.

'Must get on. Don't want to go and join them, do we?' said Mr Semple. This was a creepy statement.

'No, of course,' I said, looking at my instruments. Then I saw Mr Semple fingering his crowbar. Neil had left him armed with about every murder weapon known to man. My mind raced. I was in the middle of nowhere with some people involved in what could only be described as a bizarre activity. I didn't know anything about them. They could be very unbalanced. Goodness, I thought, they could be psychotics; Neil has twigged and made a runner. If he's getting the police, he had better be quick.

'I suppose …' I said. It had gone very quiet.

'Yes?' said Mr Semple, by now obviously brandishing his crowbar.

'Ah, your collar is wrong Richard. Before we do something reckless or which we might regret, let me…' Mrs Semple took a pace toward me to correct my wayward dress.

I jumped up, tried to lean back and coughed. She grabbed my collar forcefully and corrected it. Oh boy, what have I got myself in to? I thought.

Just then Neil returned. 'Sorted it!' he said, and he beamed. I couldn't work out if he had just phoned the police to report some psychotics or had just gone for a pee. 'Come on, Richard. Watch my back for midges or anything else and we'll complete this.'

We bent down and took the samples. Out of the corner of my eye I watched the samples. Nothing happened.

'That's fine,' Mrs Semple said. 'My husband will complete the tidying up. You had better make sure the samples meet the courier. Here is the cash you needed.' She handed Neil the agreed sum. I saw Neil was impressed by her businesslike attitude.

'Thank you. Well, good luck,' he said with a slight smile.

'Thank you, Mr Morrison and Mr Jones.' We bowed at each other and left.

'Wow!' I said. I nestled into the car seat. Malc breathed down my ear again. Compared to the previous hour his breath was vibrant with life and warmth. 'Neil, why did you leave me? You know, you really scared me! I didn't know what the hell was going on. I didn't like being left in yon gloom with that twa.'

'Oh, I never thought of that!' He laughed. 'Your imagination is far too active. I just remembered I hadn't let Malc out at lunch. It was he that needed a pee. Otherwise I thought your seat might get wet.'

'So, you mean while I was worried that you had left me with an unbalanced couple armed with all the classic murder weapons – jemmy, crowbar, chisel, hammer, never mind all our vet knives – you were taking a relaxed time off giving your dog a pee!'

'That's just about it,' replied Neil. 'Your imagination is too active, I tell you. I'm more balanced than you. No, I was only upset when Mrs Semple started bellowing. I know she didn't want to go through the whole exercise only to end up with the clone of a Banffshire midge, but there was no need for that kind of scene, quite uncalled for.'

'You weren't alone with them. I was. Besides, they are hardly normal are they?' I asked

'Is anyone?' Neil frowned. 'No, I knew them from long before. There are many crazier than them.'

To my surprise we returned to find the courier waiting for us. He had come a day early for efficiency and also to give himself time to find us in this part of Britain. I packaged up the samples and handed them to him.

'How did you get on?' asked Leasden.

'Och,' said Neil disgruntled. 'I feel I've gone back a century or so to the join the practice of the Edinburgh doctors Burke and Hare. But then I suppose it had to be done.'

'Oh, I think you're wrong, completely wrong.' Leasden examined us. 'You know, you two are at the forefront of science.' Neil and I looked at each other in surprise. Leasden continued, 'I had nothing better to do this afternoon so I read through some recent scientific journals. Let me quote you from the latest *Science America* in which MIT Professor John Jelgo said: "We are soon going to be able to clone a dog. It's only a matter of time. Working alongside us are private companies storing the DNA of dogs that have died. It may be possible that before fifty years are up to produce clones of these past creatures. Both we and they are at the cutting edge of modern science and technology." End quotes. So I bow to you Neil and Richard.' Here Leasden gave a small bow. 'My apologies for not taking you seriously. You are, I quote, "At the cutting edge".'

Chapter Seventeen
A Herculean Task

It was 7.15 am and the phone rang. I put down my cup of tea.

'Hello?' I said. Sometimes in the morning I was less open.

'Aye, hello, Richard. Alistair Gowan here.' The voice knew me.

'Oh, hello, Alistair. Quite bright morning so far,' I let on.

'Aye, it's no bad,' Alistair said. 'It would be better if it was colder and dryer. Still, can't complain.'

'That's true,' I concurred.

'Tell you why I am phoning,' Alistair went on, 'I have cow calving. I've her tied up and put my hand in. I am almost sure it's twins. I could have a go myself, but might make a heiter of it. I'd prefer you come out.'

'Fair enough,' I said. 'I'll come out now.'

'Aye, I'll see you.'

I told Jill I was off. Ten minutes later I turned into the farm. The building where most of the calving occurred was round the back.I drove round and was confronted by three generations of Gowans. I smiled. The reception committee might be unsettling to some but these were family farmers through and through. They would be shy to call themselves professionals, but that was exactly what they were.

'Aye, aye, aye!' I got out and almost bowed at the three in Japanese fashion. We went into the low building. The cow was tied to a post at a gate corner. I knew hundreds of cows had been calved here over decades. There was a rhythm and certainty in their practice which was excellent. It was a buffer against the unexpected nature of calvings. I had my PD gown on and felt inside. Sure enough, there were twins.

'Well, thank you,' I said, 'for not messing about with it. In theory you have made my job much easier because the water bags haven't burst.'

'Oh,' Alistair appeared surprised.

'Well,' I continued, 'if I break one water bag only one animal will be in it. So that saves me the bother of unravelling the legs and so on.'

'Oh, I understand that from the lambings I do,' chipped in Derek.

I broke one of the membranes and chased after the legs of the calf. Soon I had them on in spite of the calf jumping around a bit. I gave the ropes to Derek and Alistair. As they pulled I pushed the other calf back. The calf we wanted engaged into the pelvis. We quickly prepared a calving machine and had the calf out. We hung it on the gate. Soon it was breathing.

'We'd better get on with the next one,' I said. 'I've lost the second sometimes by being too slow.'

They knew what I meant, so with alacrity we found the legs of the other and pulled it out. There – we had twins alive. It was a nice start to the day. I made my goodbyes and headed to the practice. I turned into the car park to see Leasden in conversation with a farmer by a small trailer. I went in the back and found Neil opening letters.

'Oh, hello, Richard,' he said. 'Anne had to go out to a calving as well, so I'll start the small animals.'

Neil peered out through the louvres at Leasden and the farmer deep in conversation.

'I think, Richard, you should go out and see what your young friend is up to with Mr Duff. The conversation is animated.'

Acting on this suggestion, I ambled out. The conversation was more of an argument than anything else. I decided to butt in.

'Morning, Leasden. Hello, Mr Duff – what's up?'

Before I got an answer Leasden laid in. 'He's just brought an animal here to have it shot. He could have done it on the farm, save the poor creature the drive. He just wants you to shoot it.'

'No! Your friend, Mr Jones, is foo,' replied Mr Duff angrily. 'I want you to *shew* it! Jesus. Why don't they stay down south?'

I peered over the door of the trailer and saw a ewe lying down with a small vaginal prolapse at her backside. It began to make sense.

'Leasden,' I explained, 'all he wants me to do is to stitch it up.

To sew it. It has a small vaginal prolapse. This sometimes occurs near the end of pregnancy. "Foo", by the way, means he thinks you've been drinking! Tell you what, come and give me a hand to get some kit. Mr Duff, you just set her up and I'll be back in a minity.'

I explained to Leasden that Doric had some words which could be easily mistaken.

'Don't worry, it took me about six months to become proficient at understanding it. I would never try and speak it. In fact, Cantonese is about the same level. If you don't hit the tone dead right it's appalling to hear. So I don't even try unless at the request of my north-east relatives when they want me to make a fool of me for their amusement. Honestly, it's painful to hear me speak Doric. It is like someone speaking the Queen's English after elocution lessons. So don't worry: you were already in a minefield. Anyway, let us get on.'

We trooped back to the trailer. I got in and while Mr Duff held the cow I stitched her up after replacing the prolapse. I discussed the management with Mr Duff.

'That was interesting,' said Leasden.

Anne swept by in her car. She got out and we could see her face smeared with blood. Without a word she went in. We followed and tidied up our stuff. Once back in the office, we found Anne and Neil discussing what had happened.

'It was quite a stiff calving,' explained Anne. 'Eventually I got it out. In fact the last part came too easily. I placed the calf behind me and turned round to check her, only to find the whole womb running out. It just lay in a heap in front of me.'

'Nasty!' Neil commiserated. 'That's about the nastiest thing that can happen to anyone.'

'Quite,' said Anne. 'You've done all the work and just pulled out a calf. You're hot and puffed. You think you've finished the job and – bang!'

'You have to start all over again,' said Neil. 'And it's bloody hard work. No, it's awful. Rates up there with finding a twist or calving a cow for half an hour and then finding you've misjudged it and you have to do a Caesar after all. Not very pretty. But you managed okay?'

'Yes, they'll be fine. Once we had levered her up into a suitable position we got going again and had it all back. She looks bright enough. Anyway, if you don't mind,' said Anne, 'I'll go and tidy up at home. I'll be back as soon as possible.'

Leaden took me aside. 'I'd like to know more about prolapses. Are we likely to see one?'

'Well, we don't exactly go out searching for them,' I said, bemused. 'In fact they're quite rare. Much less than one per cent of all calvings. We've been doing a bit of research on them. It is pot luck whether you see one or not.'

'Then could you tell me about them?' He saw my doubtful glance. 'I'm serious. We could have lunch at the Gordon Arms and you could tell me all that you know. I could pass some of the information on to my niece.' This seemed a little tortuous, but it didn't pay to cross Leasden in earnest, and besides, he had an elephantine memory.

'Fine, then,' I concurred. 'The Gordon Arms it is.'

Three hours later we found ourselves in the upper room at the Gordon Arms. We had a table by the window. This gave a fine view of the whole square of Inverden. A statue of a past Gordon peer stood just off centre: he had crooked his elbow for the pose and some joker had recently placed an empty whisky bottle into his hand. He appeared to be extolling the virtues of drink. Apart from that hint of raffishness the square was as neat and well set as any Scottish town.

'Now tell me about uterine prolapses in cattle.' Leasden brought me back to the point in question. 'I'd like to know the A to Z from your viewpoint.'

I raised my eyebrows. 'Well, if the old boy wanted it he was going to get it now. Then out of courtesy I thought I would confirm his request.

'Are you sure? It could be a lengthy lecture…'

'Yes, yes, go on.'

I viewed the scene outside, gazed into the distance and remembered past cases. 'You know, even in the depths of the foot and mouth crisis, farmers still called us out to attend cows that had prolapsed just after calving. This is simply because it was one of the few things they can rarely do by themselves. They value the labour, expertise and experience a vet can bring to the situation. I had a break this morning so I nipped home and took out these old photos: my first prolapse, I was a student then.'

I handed these to Leasden, who examined them closely.

'My first prolapse was recorded in 1978. You can see the vet in charge, Sam, and the other student, Norman. Two matters stand out from the photos: first the well-muscled student hints at the necessity of possessing stamina and of applying a considerable amount of force when replacing a womb. Second, the sight of Sam trying to clean himself up, *après*-prolapse, in the nearby duck pond reminds me that the presence of suitable and adequate cleansing facilities has always been a bit a of a hit-and-miss affair on many UK farms. Note that we also seemed to be enjoying ourselves.'

'He has just been given a big puddle to wash in?' Leaden held the photo up in surprise. I moved on.

'One of my earliest memories as a recently qualified graduate was when I was sent out one evening to attend a Friesian cow that had prolapsed. I was doing a respectable sixty-five to seventy mph when a silver-blue Fuego shot past me, throwing up a terrific plume of spray. Funny, I thought, that looks awfully like Malcolm (the senior partner). I wonder what else he's been called out to … In the countryside you recognise individual people not only by their faces but also by their clothes, gait or car. Because of the spray I hadn't been able to confirm the number plate, but it had looked like Malcolm in a terrible hurry. I arrived at the farm to find Malcolm about to help the cow. Seeing my surprise he said, "Hello, Richard, I thought I'd just come and give a hand."

'So we set to. The prolapse was enormous. Some dairy cows are able to exteriorise the most gigantic uterus. After much huffing and puffing and the use of fists we had it all back. Malcolm gave it substantial supportive therapy. Away from the others in the dairy's washroom I thanked him and observed it appeared to go quite smoothly.

"Yes, it went well. But I know this farm; she may well be dead in a couple of days. It's odd, but for some reason which we can't discover, a lot of his don't make it. On a different farm that cow would definitely live. Still, I came because I suddenly remembered the track record of this place. I wasn't going to have a farmer lose confidence in you when it was something outside your control – and besides, they are big prolapses. Bye-bye." He leapt in his car and drove away to resume his night off duty.

'You see, in a few short sentences Malcolm had amazed me. He had rushed out to defend me, risk some of his own reputation, and tell me the grim reality. You would be wrong if you thought he was worried about losing a client. That had not been his motive; he had seen a bigger picture. The cow did die.'

'Amazing that,' commented Leasden. 'He certainly cared for the younger vet. I hope my niece is in with someone similar.'

'If it's any help, Leasden,' I went on, 'I have come up with ten golden rules for prolpases. They are not commandments; but they do help and put it into perspective. I could pass those on.'

'Why not?'

I saw his face concentrate. I paused, thinking that he would probably memorise every word. I wished I had a brain like that.

'One: once you arrive on a farm you cannot leave until there has been a resolution one way or the other. This is a matter of life and death, and also at stake is the future of the calf. To request assistance if you have good cause, for example only an eighty-year-old farmer helping with the labour, is a rational approach.

'Two: the job is hard work, messy, and on occasion a little risky. Ensure that there is hot water at home for a shower. Half the time you will need it.

'Three: no single technique is guaranteed to succeed in every case. This is because the type of uterine prolapse, location, available labour, and water supply etc. varies enormously.

'Four: you have to be well drilled in a set technique which you are confident with. Yet you must also be competent to use many different techniques which you are not familiar with.

'Five: it is crucial, whatever technique you use, to ensure that you have created a set of circumstances in which gravity is going to aid your efforts to replace the womb. Only the young and very fit can replace a womb against a slope; your niece will not be young for ever, so she must learn a technique that has gravity as an assistant.

'Six: the mortality rate of *all* uterine prolpasess that your niece will attend is usually *above* that of Caesarian sections. A possible figure would be that at least one in fourteen die. "Death" includes not being alive one month after the event. To my mind this is a realistic figure. Nineteen times out of twenty her judgement will be correct about the prognosis. However, at least one in twenty cases will unexpectedly and often dramatically survive or die in spite of her reasoned prognosis.

'Seven: she should use fists. Be careful that neither you or anyone helping ever pushes in such a manner that a finger rips through the endometrium. On rare occasions you can push with fingers – but "ca' canny". Amazingly, one can lose the odd cotyledon and get away with it, but this should not be a matter of routine.

'Eight: calcium is always required. The debate is whether before or after. The calcium does assist in shrinking the womb (as does sugar). It will also strengthen the cow in expelling the uterus while you are replacing it.

'Nine: it is worth placing a stitch across the vulval lips once the prolapse is replaced. The main merit of doing this is that it will slow down or partially stop any prolapse which is about to come out again. This buys you some time and reduces the possibility of severe shock. The vet must make very effort to thoroughly invert the womb. If your niece is short-armed (like me), then use a bottle – preferably a hock bottle – to form a blunt extension of the arm. Both parts of the womb should be inverted. Failure to do this greatly increases the risk of the womb reappearing.'

'Ten: approximately one in thirty wombs will come out again, even if correctly replaced. The two common causes are unreasonable continuous pressing by the cow, or uncorrected hypocalcaemia. Epidurals may not always halt these contractions: extra calcium should be given if milk fever is suspected. The use of water to fill the womb once replaced is usually very effective in these situations. However, it may not be available. I hope that is of some use.'

'Oh yes,' said Leasden. 'It will certainly help. The photos show that it is an enormous thing about the size of four or six rugby balls that you are trying to replace back through a relatively small hole. Tricky, isn't it?'

'Yes, I think so. Now, prolapse cases have a variable result. Some die unexpectedly, others live – to your surprise – so I might tell you of a couple of incidents.'

'Fire away.' Leasden seemed to be gobbling it up.

'There comes a time in some prolapse cases when you know the game is up and she is about to die. Usually in this dramatic scene the gums are as white as a sheet and the cow goes through some fairly distressing agonal gasps as she slips away. It is a test to a vet how he handles this situation, which is beyond his control. It is caused by the sporadic and insoluble problem of internal bleeding. I remember my first such occasion: the prolapse had been easily replaced, with the cow tied up in her own stall. She had stood still like a guardsman on parade. It was dusk; I had been invited in for a cup of tea by the farmer whereupon he let out the significant phrase: "It's good to get a vet out, particularly when he can save a beast like yon."' I halted and looked out again over at the square.

'Now I'm older and wiser, I realise the alarm bells should have rung. But I was young and green in judgement and so I warmed to the compliment. Tea and cakes finished, we all trooped out to have one final look. As we went in the byre we saw the cow stumbling, trying to keep to her feet. Obviously she was fainting. We desperately tried to help her but within two minutes she was dead. In the darkness I left, stunned.'

'Nasty,' said Leasden with feeling.

'Nowadays I quickly tell the farmer what is about to occur if I see it coming. Even now I notice how hard it is for all of us to grasp the truth of what is happening. In my opinion it is quite acceptable for the air to go blue and for any farmer to go for a walk.' Leasden nodded.

'Still, there is a flip side. This is what happened to Eddy. He called me out to a heifer once and I was just about to set to when he spoke to me. At the time it was like hearing an oracle,' I continued.

'"Wait, I would save your energy!" Eddy had said to me as I was about to replace the prolapse. I stopped and saw what he meant. The heifer was almost motionless. Very rarely, she gave a small breath. Eddy leant against the small heifer, steadying her,

271

and waited for the inevitable, which over sixty years of farming had taught him would come. So I just sat down on my ankles behind her. I had noticed that the vaginal mucus membranes were very pale. We looked down from the grassy knoll at the river glinting in the sunshine about three hundred yards away. It was a truly lovely morning.

'Two minutes and three breaths later I looked at Eddy.

'"She's not living and she's not dying either. I think I'll just get on with it," I said. As her head was downhill and she was behaving like an animal under extreme anaesthesia, the womb was easily replaced.

'"I'll just give her a couple of jabs," I said. I knew he would rightly think I was taking advantage of him if I filled her full of drugs with her so close to death. Even so I mixed some Betsolan with Hexasol in one syringe and put calcium IV in with the other needle. I will charge him for the Betsolan if she lives, I reasoned. We rotated her so her head was facing up the hill to reduce the risk of choke or bloat and left her. Halfway across the field I looked round to see her still comatose, her chin resting on the ground surrounded by the most idyllic rural scene.

'We hardly said anything to each other walking across the park.

'"Well, we'll see," I said as I got in my car, "Please give me a phone either way... see you." And off I went.'

'And?' Leasden asked.

'Next day Eddy phoned to say she was fine. Halfway through the afternoon she had risen and slowly gone to the river to drink. She was not 100% but was definitely on the mend, eating and so on. This goes to show that you can always get an odd surprise with this condition.'

'But it is rare?' asked Leasden.

'Well, yes and no. Two of the more surprising ones I remember happened at one farm. Chris called me out to a prolapse. When I arrived we scoured the field for the cow; she must have moved after he phoned. Eventually we saw a small dot hard against the fence way down at the bottom of the field. It was very early in the morning and the Land Rover was slipping a bit on the dew-soaked grass. When we arrived we found her in an impossible situation at the bottom of a slope, with the fence strainers stopping her moving further down a steep precipice into a rugged pine forest. She was very dull and depressed. The calf was wandering around bawling but the cow took no notice.

"'We'll have to move her, Chris,'" I had told him. "I can't push a prolapse as big as this up a hill." She was a big cow and try as we could we were unable shift her into any sensible position. All the time she was looking worse and worse. So with little to lose, we tied her forelegs to the rear of the Rover to pull her off the fence and up the hill. I was going to follow up behind supporting the womb in a fertiliser bag but Chris wouldn't have it. He was scared the Land Rover would slip on the dew and then the cow and more would end up on me. Instead, we agreed to put a halter on her head and I would pull on that too. Up we went, and I could just see the large prolapse going bump-bump over the grass! It was all a bit bizarre. After forty yards the slope levelled a bit, so we turned the Land Rover round and halted her on this relatively flat surface. Then we had a terrible time steadying her onto her brisket. There was nothing flat or level and the cow behaved like a gigantic sack of potatoes. Finally, with her in sternal recumbency, I began to attempt to put the womb back. Even with a completely comatose cow it surprised me in this case how much effort was required. Finally it was in. I gave her calcium, Hexasol and some Betsolan.

"'Well, we will surely see,'" I had said grimly.

"'Oh, I don't know, I've seen much worse,'" said Chris. "She has a chance." And he was right. She did make it.'

'Oh well, I suppose if you're in with a chance you are in with a chance,' said Leasden optomistically.

'Yes, it is so. The incident Chris was referring to had occurred three years previously. Early one morning the senior partner, Eric Strachan, had been called to a cow that had prolapsed in a similar field. However, this time the cow was very bright, alert and able to run. Eric and Chris arrived in the field to see the cow moving quite fast with the womb going slap-slap-slap against her hind quarters. They tried desperately not to chase her or upset her, but with no success. She shot up the hill and after a short sprint the whole womb ruptured near the cervix and fell off. She went a little further and lay down but kept her head up. Eric prodded the womb at his feet and left, saying there was nothing practical he could do, just leave her alone. She should faint and pass away in a few minutes.

'At lunchtime Chris phoned asking to speak to Eric. Eric took the phone with few premonitions.

'"What am I to do about my cow, Eric? She is in exactly the same position lying head up!" Eric was incredulous and asked Chris if he was winding him up.

'"No," said Chris.

'"Well, you had better just leave her. If you move her now the bleeding could start. Tomorrow, if she's alive, move her off the hill slowly and get her inside and I'll give you something for her."

'She did live, and I recall seeing her indoors. She appeared a little highly strung but otherwise normal.

'"Fancy PDing her?" Chris had asked me.'

'Incredible!' said Leasden

'Oh, I know, and no one believes us, even with at least three witnesses. That factual account is condemned to the realms of fiction. A bizarre world we live in, isn't it?' I raised my eyes. 'Now, I've written down here on this piece of paper exactly what I do for technique. You can pass it on to your niece. It's not written in tablets of stone. As I said, she has to find a technique and method she is comfortable with. However, I will also tell you of one or two unconventional ways.'

Leasden took the notes, murmuring thanks.

'The hosepipe: once inverted, the womb can be filled with water using a hose and a generous flow of water. You just attach a pipe up her reproductive tract and inflate it with cold water. In the standing cow this effectively guarantees that the womb will not reappear. If the water is cold the cow trembles in an unnerving way, but they seem to be able to take a large volume. On one occasion a farmer called me to a prolapse which had come out after he had replaced it. The cow was tied in the stall and the womb was easily replaced. But I did notice that she was continuously pressing.

'I put a stitch on her and gave an epidural and calcium. On my arrival back at the practice the phone rang to inform me that the womb was out again. Back I went. I could now clearly see that this cow had one ambition in life: to continuously strain. It appeared to be psychological. Once again I put the womb in. Farmer and I discussed the situation with our hands and a bottle inside her, desperately trying to stop the fourth coming. I asked for a hosepipe and ditched the bottle. We secured the pipe between and beyond our "indwelling hands", while the cow strained vigorously as though she still had a large calf to deliver.

'I can only guess at the volumes, but I think in any one minute we filled her with more than four gallons of water, and she by one or two heaves expelled more than three gallons. The farmer's wife was standing to one side and said it look like a scene from a maritime disaster movie! Gallons of water shot over our heads and coursed down the inside of our clothes. All the time we were desperately trying to plug this gap in the cow's rear. Except for the fact it was the cow's life at stake, the lady said it was the funniest thing she had seen in a long time... Eventually, as the minutes went by, the cow's straining reduced as she filled up. Finally she stopped. Very gingerly we tried to ascertain how much water was in her. It seemed a large loch. Her belly was large and rounded. Quietly, we left her standing. He told me later she recovered uneventfully – bar the fact that she didn't drink for the first two days!

'Next, the loader: it is not my favourite aid. However, I have been known to use it. When the farmer has it to hand and is keen and experienced in its use, it can seem churlish to refuse. But your niece must be careful. Ropes are tied around the hocks and the cow is slowly and carefully lifted vertically. Great care must be taken not to have any twist on the sacroiliac junction. All the ropes must be secure. There must be no sudden movement which could endanger the cow and the operators. Once lifted, it is relatively easy to replace the womb.

'Finally, the mound: at the far end of my father-in-law's cow byre in Followsters there is large mound of impacted earth. It is about the size and shape of a very large anthill. Above it is a medicine cabinet, which was always well managed but undocumented, and above that under the eaves was hidden a bottle of whisky. That was for beast and man – in that order of priority. I asked him the purpose of the mound. He said in previous days if a cow had a prolapse they would manhandle the cow to this mound. In those days there was more labour on farms and closer neighbours to help. At the mound they would pull the cow down on to it with her hips stuck on the slope and the head on the byre floor. Thus positioned, it was easy with the rear pointing upwards for them to replace the womb themselves. The same principle applies today. If there is a mound or hillock which you can use quickly, then use it. And so I rest my case.'

'Well,' said Leasden, 'I can't but thank you. It has been very informative and I am sure it will help my niece. I myself have also learnt a thing or two.'

We returned to the day's labours.

Chapter Eighteen
Endgame

It was Saturday morning. I walked into the lab to find Neil sharpening a large post-mortem knife.

'Morning, Neil,' I greeted him. 'Who's that for?' I wondered if he was off to post-mortem a beast.

'I haven't decided yet,' was the ambiguous reply. I headed off for the office.

'Is Neil okay?' I asked June.

'Oh, as ever,' she said.

I had only to work the morning. Once that was complete I had the day free. A weight would lift from my shoulders while the vet on duty had to carry on with all the strain.

We soon finished the small animal work. Leasden came in while Neil went off to vaccinate a horse. There was little happening, so I decided to take a walk to the square to check out something at the newsagent's. As I came by I saw a shape I recognised staring in at one of the windows. It was James, the chemistry teacher from Norbury. I came slowly up to him and confirmed my first guess.

'Oh, hello, James. We met before at my aunt's in Norbury. What brings you up here?'

James started and then regained his composure.

'Richard, Richard – of course, how nice to see you,' he said breathlessly. 'Far cry from Norbury in every way. I am *en passant*. Driving up to see an aunt, would you believe, in Tain. I stopped off for a break. Nice town here.'

'Yes, it is pleasant here,' I replied. 'Still, the cold weather seems to limit the number of folk up here.'

'It is a bit chilly, I must admit.' James folded his hands.

'If you need a break why not come back to my practice? Have a cup of coffee ... warm you up, set you on your way. You'd never

believe it but there's someone else from Norbury here too:
Leasden.'

'Ah, really, Claude… what a surprise!' This seemed a little
forced. Perhaps he and Leasden did not see eye to eye.

'He's not too bad, you know, particularly when he is on my
patch,' I said.

'I think I'll have to give it a miss, you know,' he said.

'And my aunt – have you seen my aunt recently?' I asked.

'Recently, recently …' he was playing with the word. 'Yes. Yes,
I have. She seemed in fine form, quite bubbly actually.'

'Oh, that's good,' I said. 'I did enjoy my time down there.'

'Yes, your aunt is a…' he paused, 'a wonderful creature. So
kind so thoughtful.' He had gone a little pink.

'Yes, she was always very kind to me,' I said.

'Look, Richard. Humble apologies and all that, but I really
have to go and dash on north.' With that he disappeared.

Bemused, I went back to the practice.

'I sent Leasden home,' explained June. 'There are no small
animal appointments apart from removing stitches and a couple of
boosters. I hope you don't mind.'

'No, June, it makes absolute sense,' I replied.

Time flew, and soon I found myself driving down the hill to
home. There was always a terrific sense of freedom at that
moment. The weight of being on call lifted, the day still with
many hours to go for anything I pleased to do, and all of Sunday
free to look forward to.

I walked into the kitchen. To my surprise, I found Aunt Sarah
sitting at the kitchen table. Her dark hair contrasted with her light
jacket top. As always, she was immaculately turned out. She
smiled at me and then looked down at the tabletop. It was quite
unlike her to appear so nervous.

'Hello, Aunt Sarah,' I said. 'This is a surprise, a nice surprise.
What brings you here?'

Jill was standing by behind Aunt Sarah. For some reason my
wife was smiling broadly.

'Aunt Sarah has an announcement. She has had some good
luck!' Jill beamed at me. 'We could even put something on ice to
drink.'

'Well, no need to come all this way to make an announcement or if you have had some good luck, great! But you could have easily picked up the phone.'

'No, you don't get it, Richard,' said Jill. At that point I saw Aunt Sarah look a little nervous. 'Aunt Sarah is most likely about to be engaged! Isn't that terrific?'

'Why, yes, of course.' I was bemused. 'Great! Do I know the lucky man?'

'You should do,' hinted Jill, 'you likely saw him today.'

'Oh, oh – James, the teacher at college!' The penny had suddenly dropped. I met him before at Norbury and today I had seen him in the square here in Inverden. He had kept on speaking about Aunt Sarah. 'Well now, that is a good choice. Thoroughly good man. Mind you he appeared nervous too. Big decision and all that, Aunt Sarah, but you shouldn't be so uptight.'

Aunt Sarah swallowed smiled forcefully and looked up at Jill.

'No, Richard. Wrong man!' A little urgency crept in to Jill's voice. 'James only drove Aunt Sarah up here. It is *Claude Leasden* she is intending to be engaged to. Isn't that marvellous?'

There was a long silence and then I exploded.

'Marvellous? *Marvellous? I think she's mad!*' I said directly at Jill.

Jill's eyes lit up as though aflame. Aunt Sarah's head bent down and she sobbed.

'I knew it,' Aunt Sarah cried. 'I knew this was a bad luck!'

'Richard,' hissed Jill. 'I despise you. Have you no consideration for anyone else? Do you only think about your own feelings? Does anybody else have feelings? Good God, you are the most harmful brute I have ever known.'

'No, he's okay,' interjected Aunt Sarah. She began to wipe her tears away with her hair. Her Adam's apple went up and down a couple of times and she took a deep breath. 'Perhaps he's right. Maybe it would be no good. How could I ever ever expect you two to get on? It was hopeless. At least I tried.'

'Tried?' I asked.

'Yes, she did,' concurred Jill. 'In fact she had a good plan, a sort of agreement.' I was obviously confused. I shrugged at Jill with my eyes wide open.

'Did or did you not speak with Claude Leasden,' asked Jill, 'when he went out seeing practice with you?'

'Of course I spoke with him,' I replied testily. 'We were together for many days.'

'Did or did you not have any serious arguments with him,' she continued, 'during this period of seeing practice?' I could sense the lawyer's hat had been placed on.

'No,' I responded. 'We had no serious disagreements. None that I can recollect, anyway.'

'Did or did you not have three or more rational discussions with Claude?' she then asked. I could now deduce that her lawyer's hat had been secured firmly. Aunt Sarah just stared at me. Tears had dried on her cheeks.

'Yes,' I replied. 'He seemed pretty reasonable. In fact, from time to time we got on quite well with each other. But then I can get on with most folk.'

'See!' said Jill, looking at Aunt Sarah. 'He has managed to do what he said he would. I think you should go ahead. He—' she nodded in my direction— 'will have to come round to it.'

'*What* did he manage to do?' I asked angrily.

'Richard, stop being so loud,' urged Jill. 'She was only trying to be reasonable. Tell him, Sarah. I thought it was a good idea.'

Aunt Sarah started very slowly. 'Well, it goes like this, Richard. In China where I come from we have great respect for the family. We try not to hurt other members of the family. So after Claude and I started going out I realised there might be trouble. I remembered about you and Classics. I was in the town during the years when you were at school and I had worked out that it was Claude that you did not get on with.' She paused.

'Go on,' I said dully.

'When you came down for that weekend my fears were confirmed. You remember – you came back in a mood after you had met Claude at the market.'

'Yes, I remember,' I said.

'So I met up with Claude later. I told him I had doubts about our friendship going deeper because it would be a problem with my favourite relative and possibly the rest of the family.'

'Oh, Aunt Sarah!' I said in exasperation.

'Anyway, at least I wanted to know that you two could talk to each other and be civilised. And I told Claude that. He was a little surprised but then he said it was most important that I was happy and content in my own mind and that I knew I was doing the right thing.'

'Very wise,' said Jill.

'So I said to Claude that if he could have at least three reasonable conversations with you then I would consider us making a go of it.'

'Three reasonable conversations?' I said. 'I don't believe it! So that's why he kept at me! He wanted to know about the A to Z of prolapses because of Aunt Sarah – and to get in with her. He wanted to know about the Competition Commission for the same reason. I bet the recidivist doesn't even have a niece who is a vet!' I bellowed.

'He has. We met. She lives,' retorted Jill

'Does she?' I barked.

'She is a nice, quiet and polite veterinary surgeon.' Jill fixed on me. The implicit criticism was scathing.

'So! *You* were in on this?' I demanded of my wife.

'Not immediately,' she replied off-handedly. 'The day after Claude brought you home drunk and legless I phoned Aunt Sarah. My suspicions were aroused. So I asked Aunt Sarah whether this was coincidence or if something was up. Then she told me all. So I decided to help her a little. I think Claude has done very well. Not only has he had many reasonable conversations with you; he has even seen practice. And you had the temerity to drag him up a hill one night to do a Caesar. That shows some commitment.'

'I feel as though I have been made a fool of. I think that's what makes me really angry,' I said, looking at both of them.

'Ah, Richard, but for a good cause,' added Jill. 'It has only hurt your feelings. Your professional integrity is still there. And would you deny your aunt some happiness?'

'No, no, you're right, my love,' I said in a weary tone. 'Claude Leasden certainly tried damn hard. I can't take that away from him. If that shows his commitment to Aunt Sarah, well then I can't but say go on, go on! But please, do I have to be polite to him *all* the time?'

'*Richard* ...' said Jill firmly.

'I see … I do,' I smiled. 'Okay, okay, you two, you win, you win. But you can understand why I am a little angry.'

'Yes,' said Jill, 'but that is half because of the type of buddy you are. '

'And the other half?' I asked.

'Well, some of it may be due to Claude's manner,' observed Jill. 'But then, that is Aunt Sarah's joy. Just as you are, shall I say, my joy.' She gave me a fixed grin.

'Are you sure you'll be okay?' I asked Aunt Sarah.

'Yes, so long as you see my viewpoint,' said Aunt Sarah.

'Yes, yes, Aunt, I do. So long as we can draw a line under this affair I am more than happy. We'd better put something on ice after all. Where is your man anyway? Aunt Sarah? Is he walking round outside this house looking for smoke to come from a chimney?'

'No, he's upstairs,' said Jill. 'I instructed him not to come down, no matter what he heard. It's a good thing I did say that. I'll get him.' She ran down the corridor. 'Claude, Claude it's agreed! All will be well. Come down now at once!'

I saw Leasden come down. He was walking on his toes.

'You know the story?' he asked nervously.

'I do. Congratulations! After what you've done you deserve the best luck. No need to come out with me again.' I moved forward and shook his hand. He grasped it firmly.

'Well, I am relieved.' He looked down at his toes and then up. 'I do have a niece. That was true. Now I know it's a tough job she succeeds in.'

Aunt Sarah stood up and grabbed his hand. It was obvious that they were very much in love.

Jill came back and passed me a bottle of champagne to open. I soon filled four glasses.

'Well, Claude, Sarah …' I stood up, pompously commencing a speech. 'I think this was an unconventional set of proceeding circumstances to an engagement. Perhaps there were extraordinary and extenuating circumstances. Nevertheless, you have coped marvellously.' Before I could get any further I felt a kick on my shin. Blow the lawyer, I thought. They speak enough when they want to. I carried on. 'This brings me to wish you the best in the future. I am sure you care for each other very much. And I fully expect you to be much happier than Jill and I have been as a married couple—' At this point I felt my toe being ground into the floor. I sucked in my breath. 'I wish you could be much happier than Jill and I as a married couple – if that were possible – something which I doubt!'

Laughter all round. 'I propose a toast to the wedding of Sarah and Claude... soon may it be.' Glasses were clinked and wine sipped religiously.

'Wait till I get my hands on you in bed,' whispered my spouse.

'I'll be ready for you, woman,' I muttered back.

'I have to reply to such kind words,' murmured Leasden, faining deafness. Aunt Sarah was by now leaning on his shoulder. 'I have a simple toast as a peace offering. I propose to the person I have had the pleasure of accompanying round some farms; to Richard. In my opinion he is *A Classical Vet in Modern Times*.'

Even Jill was impressed; either by the diplomacy, or else the sentiment moved her. She raised her glass and said, 'I can drink to that ... *A Classical Vet in Modern Times*.'

Postscript
By Edward Jones

Pro captu lectoris habent sua fata libelli – The fate of books depends on the capacity of the reader.

Terentianus Maurus, AD 200, *De Literis Syllabis*

So Dad has at last made his peace with his Classics master. Personally, I think Mr Leasden – or Claude, as Rachel insists on calling him behind his back – is a nice kind of guy. Anyone who wants to blow up a hateful Physics teacher is well balanced as far as I am concerned. Now Dad has gone and written a book about the whole Leasden/Aunt Sarah affair: this is mega embarrassing, and I am only saved by the reduced reading appetites of my friends. There is, of course, another side to the whole story, and before everyone is convinced that Dad is *the* Classical Vet I thought I would, for money, write my side of the story.

I first realised my Dad was a vet when we lived in Hong Kong: he slept with a baby orang-utan for three nights. Before this occurrence I never realised what his occupation was. Every morning in Hong Kong my father left for work wearing smart clothes. He was a typical civil servant wearing a shirt, tie, carrying a briefcase, and travelling down to the office in Kowloon. However, this is not the case now we are back in Britain; my dad leaves for work in old shirts and trousers as he has to be prepared for the occasionally messy work he encounters on the farms he visits.

As I live in the same house as a vet, the phone is ringing constantly during the day and sometimes during the night hours. From time to time this can cause problems, as friends sometimes think they have dialled the wrong number after they hear, 'Hello, Veterinary Centre?' Another drawback of Dad being on call is that other members of the family cannot stay on the phone for a long time in case someone is trying to contact the vets. This especially affects my elder sister, because she uses the phone the most. We do have a second phone line, but this still doesn't solve the problem, as someone is usually on line and broadband hasn't reached this area yet. Although my dad rarely wakes me as he leaves on a night call, I hear about it in the morning from others members of the family, whether it was a case of staggers, a calving or a Caesar.

Occasionally my dad comes home in a bloody mess from head to toe. Mum stops him at the door and makes him strip off all his dirty clothes before he trollops around the house. This is usually because he has been to a messy calving or prolapse. His trousers are too dirty to put in the washing machine, so they are thrown into a bucket of hot soapy water and are left to soak. Now and again, shirts are completely ruined because the bloodstains are too heavy to clean. Sometimes he is so messy the shower needs to be cleaned after he has used it. Even when he comes home clean it's not unusual for him to arrive home with a musky vetty smell lingering around himself and his clothes. This is probably due to the wide variation of drugs and disinfectants he deals with on a regular basis.

While on call, my dad cannot drink any alcohol. However, he makes up for it when he is free from his veterinary duties. On his weekends off duty he plants himself on the sofa with his bottle of port and watches the Premiership contentedly. On Wednesday night after hockey practice he comes home from the pub happy and oblivious to everything – even the 'I hope you didn't drink too much' lecture from Mum.

My dad has a rather outdated fashion sense. This is worsened by the fact that he has to be prepared to be called out at any moment, and consequently is dressed for any eventuality. For this reason most of his clothes are clean but old and tattered. This causes a small problem for the teenage members of the family as some of us are embarrassed to be seen with him when he's wearing such retro items. As my dad is a vet I don't expect him to wear expensive designer labels or fashionable clothes, but I would have expected his dress code to be of a higher standard than it is currently. I don't think body warmers make neat items of dress…

In the morning Mum leaves home wearing a smart black suit and heads off to her solicitor's office job in a clean, small, nimble car. In contrast to this Dad leaves home wearing old ragged clothes and departs for work in a mud-spotted, heavy car packed to the brink with veterinary drugs and equipment. A long metal pole that spans the length of his car is also crammed in. It is a special device used for calvings. Although some parts of the car are untidy, the boot is surprisingly well ordered, with drugs and other medicines. Occasionally, my dad gives members of the family lifts to places in his car. However, these are rare, as his car has a potent smell that loiters within the compartment.

Many vets have a dog in the car; however my dad doesn't take our Golden Retriever with him anymore. His excuse is that it is 'poor biosecurity'. The actual reason is that one day a member of the family fed the dog the remains of an Indian takeaway for breakfast. At the first farm visit the dog vomited and voided all over the front seat. Ever since that event, Dad has never taken the dog to work with him again. He and a receptionist spent a very long time cleaning up all the curry smells; but the vetty smells still linger around. The in-car air-fresheners do not work very well.

My friends don't have any views on my dad being a vet. Nowadays for many teenagers being a vet is nothing special; this is true even for those who have pets like us. Besides, we don't talk much about our parents' jobs. Some of my friends' parents have long working hours, but the majority have nine-to-five jobs.

My parents are always harassing me about my homework, but recently I have found out that they also have a form of homework to do. It goes by the name of CPD. I don't know what the initials stand for, but I do know that they both have to do about twenty hours a year. Both of my parents do it in different ways. My mum takes law journals home to study and travels in to Aberdeen now and again to achieve her twenty hours of homework. My dad does his twenty hours by going to conferences and doing the required work at the office; at least, that's what he says he does. Unlike me, there doesn't seem to be anybody checking on him. He never has a veterinary magazine home. The good side to this is that, apart from when he is on duty, work doesn't affect us here at home.

After living on my grandad's beef farm for a while and seeing some of the work that my dad encounters, I have decided that my future does not lie within veterinary medicine. I have a few reasons for this; firstly I would prefer a nine-to-five job; I wouldn't like the prospect of being called out at nights. In addition to this, I also don't like the idea of driving to all the different farms over a widespread area; speaking personally I would prefer a job indoors in an office. In conclusion, it is interesting having a vet living in the same household. It is fascinating for me to find out about the great variety of work he does each day and I am glad it's him doing it and not me.

Printed in the United Kingdom
by Lightning Source UK Ltd.
104334UKS00001B/1-30